Children with Medical Complexity in the Emergency Department

Audrey Kamzan • Deepa Kulkarni
Charles A. Newcomer
Editors

Children with Medical Complexity in the Emergency Department

A Case-Based Guide

Springer

Editors
Audrey Kamzan
Pediatrics
Mattel Children's Hospital
Los Angeles, CA, USA

Deepa Kulkarni
Pediatrics
Mattel Children's Hospital
Los Angeles, CA, USA

Charles A. Newcomer
Pediatrics
Santa Barbara Cottage Hospital
Santa Barbara, CA, USA

ISBN 978-3-031-62516-9 ISBN 978-3-031-62517-6 (eBook)
https://doi.org/10.1007/978-3-031-62517-6

This Springer imprint is published by the registered company Springer Nature Switzerland AG
The registered company address is: Gewerbestrasse 11, 6330 Cham, Switzerland

Preface

As pediatric hospitalists working in a busy and complex pediatric tertiary/quaternary care center, we are frequently consulted by the emergency department to help assess and stabilize children with medical complexity (CMC). We also receive calls from emergency departments outside of our institution caring for these patients in their community emergency rooms and hoping to transfer them to a center with the proper resources and support to care for them. Over the years, we have seen over and over how critical it is that emergency care providers have a working knowledge of the principles of disease and treatment for these high risk patients. The first few hours of care are often critical and cannot always wait until the transfer to a tertiary or quaternary care center is complete. We have found that many emergency providers did not receive adequate training in the acute care of CMC and that there is a great deal of interest in better understanding how to care for this patient population.

One of us is also the parent of a child with medical complexity who has experienced first-hand the fear and anxiety families face when they bring a medically complex child into an emergency department that is unable to provide appropriate care. These challenges are big ones that require big solutions, including better integration and dissemination of medical information and broader access to specialized care for patients in underserved areas. While this text cannot solve all of these problems alone, we hope that it may be one piece of a solution by spreading information and expertise about the acute care of children with medical complexity to those on the frontlines who need it most.

Sincerely,

Los Angeles, CA, USA — Audrey Kamzan
Los Angeles, CA, USA — Deepa Kulkarni
Santa Barbara, CA, USA — Charles A. Newcomer

Contents

Introduction: Special Considerations in the Care of Children with Medical Complexity 1
Deepa Kulkarni, Audrey Kamzan, and Charles A. Newcomer

Vomiting in a Child with a Metabolic Disorder 5
Margaret Nguyen, Youngeun Park, and Yue Huang

A Patient with Leukemia and a Fever 15
Rabia Cheema, Miriam Beyder, and Camille Hamilton

A Patient with a History of Traumatic Brain Injury and Fever 25
Lucia An, Christopher J. Ferber, and Hanna Siddiqui

Cloudy Dialysate Effluent and Abdominal Pain in a Patient on Peritoneal Dialysis 35
Madison Shirkey Anderson and Rose Ayoob

Respiratory Distress in a Patient with Congenital Heart Disease 43
Megan M. McKittrick, Laura A. Maitoza, and Mai-King C. Chan

An Infant with Prolonged Fever, Splenomegaly, and Rash 55
Evan Wiley

A Child with Medical Complexity and Worsening Irritability 63
Jonathan Fliegel and Sara Liegel

Cystic Fibrosis Pulmonary Exacerbation 71
Harrison Luttrell, Jeffrey C. Winer, and Tonia E. Gardner

An Infant Born at Extreme Prematurity Presenting in Respiratory Distress 79
Alexandra Vinci, Dimpy Mody, Tuan Nguyen, and Thomas Duggan

Fever in a Patient with Short Bowel Syndrome 93
Rebecca Tenney-Soeiro and Christina Bales

A Child with Bleeding from a Tracheostomy Tube 103
James A. Lin and Alisha N. West

A Dislodged Gastrostomy Tube 115
Rena Sarhangian and Kelly Fong

A Complication of a Central Line 121
Yamini Sharma and Grace Sund

A Complication of Bladder Reconstruction 131
Elizabeth Mannino Avila, George Chiang, and Julia Beauchamp Walters

A Child with a Ventriculoperitoneal Shunt and Fever 141
Jasen Liu, Vivian Lin, Kristina Adachi, and Anthony Wang

An Adolescent with an Ostomy and Abdominal Pain 151
Marie Dawlett and Amy Gonzalez

A Patient with a Heart Transplant and Abdominal Pain 157
Helen Zhou, Majid Husain, and Juan Alejos

A Renal Transplant Recipient with Elevated Blood Pressure and Loose Stool 169
Allison E. Williams and Elizabeth Spiwak

A Patient with a Liver Transplant and Abdominal Pain 177
Stacey Stauber, Esther Jun-Ihn, and Robert Venick

Increased Ostomy Output and Fevers in a Child with Small Bowel Transplant 183
Esther Jun-Ihn, Stacey Stauber, and Robert Venick

A Complication of Polypharmacy 189
Shahram Yazdani, Pauline Yi, and Vidhi Doshi

Index 207

Introduction: Special Considerations in the Care of Children with Medical Complexity

Deepa Kulkarni, Audrey Kamzan, and Charles A. Newcomer

Children with medical complexity (CMC) make up a particularly vulnerable subset of pediatric patients. These are patients with at least one chronic medical condition that is severe or contributes to significant morbidity and/or mortality [1]. They are high utilizers of the healthcare system, often requiring several medications, technology (e.g., feeding tubes, breathing tubes, or other assistive devices), and frequent visits with medical providers. Most pediatric residency programs lack dedicated curricula focused on teaching trainees to care for these medically complex patients. Thus, much of their care is provided by highly trained pediatric subspecialists in tertiary and quaternary care centers. However, many of these centers are far from the communities in which these children and families live. Although there has been an increase in the pediatric subspecialty workforce over time, the geographic distribution still favors urban areas with millions of children residing more than 90 min from their specialty providers [2]. Some of the burden of transportation to and from these centers has been alleviated by the increase in telehealth visits with pediatric subspecialists.

However, emergency care must be available in person and nearby to ensure prompt evaluation and management of these medically fragile patients. Similar to pediatric trainees, emergency medicine trainees also lack built-in curricula focused on children with medical complexity and often do not feel confident when caring for them [3]. Despite this, emergency medicine physicians are critical to the care of these children. When children with medical complexity are acutely ill, they are highly likely to present to an emergency department (ED) within their community,

D. Kulkarni (✉) · A. Kamzan
Department of Pediatrics, UCLA Mattel Children's Hospital, Los Angeles, CA, USA
e-mail: dkulkarni@mednet.ucla.edu; akamzan@mednet.ucla.edu

C. A. Newcomer
Department of Pediatrics, Santa Barbara Cottage Hospital, Santa Barbara, CA, USA
e-mail: cnewcome@sbch.org

A. Kamzan et al. (eds.), *Children with Medical Complexity in the Emergency Department*, https://doi.org/10.1007/978-3-031-62517-6_1

regardless of whether they are equipped with pediatric emergency medicine physicians or other pediatric subspecialists. Studies show that while the patient population seen in pediatric EDs tends to be more complex, children with complex medical conditions are overall much more likely to receive care in a general ED than in a pediatric ED [4].

It is therefore essential that providers in all settings, including the community, have the knowledge to care for these patients while awaiting recommendations from or transfer to a pediatric center. When that is not the case, patients and families suffer. Parents of CMC have reported feelings of anxiety and frustration related to ED visits. They describe extensive wait times, communication gaps within provider teams and between providers and families, and the burdensome need to constantly explain their child's condition [5]. Families experience these challenges frequently due to their child's fragility and complexity and the continual need for care. Studies show that they are less satisfied than parents of children with no special healthcare needs. They rate their child's care lower when asked if doctors listen to them, explain things easily, show respect, and spend enough time with them [6]. The difficulties these families face when they seek acute care only add to the many challenges they deal with when navigating the healthcare system. It is perhaps then not surprising that among all parents, those with CMC are the most likely to report suboptimal mental health [7].

Solutions have been proposed to ease transitions between hospital sites and ensure safe care for children with medical complexity across settings. One such solution is the implementation of emergency information forms (EIFs), also known as "pediatric passports," a handoff document that providers can either upload to the electronic health record or provide in hard copy to families. These documents contain critical information such as a list of medical problems, allergies, medical history and diagnoses, contact information for the patient's primary medical team, and important action items during times of illness. EIFs are intended both to better prepare and engage the family in the patients' care and to provide clear information to new providers when these patients present for acute care. Such tools are particularly useful when children present to institutions less familiar with the patients or their rare disease processes. EIFs have been found to enhance patient and family perception of communication between and within medical teams. This effect has also been found in the use of pediatric passports among families who are primarily Spanish-speaking, who are particularly vulnerable to adverse events and miscommunication [8]. Qualitative studies have also demonstrated that providers and caregivers of CMC see EIFs as an effective way to mitigate some of the challenges of seeking emergency care for CMC [9]. The American College of Emergency Physicians and the American Academy of Pediatrics have both released policy statements supporting the use of EIFs whenever possible for children with medical complexity [10, 11]. Recommendations in these policy statements include designating medical home or primary care providers as those best equipped to prepare EIFs and that they should be reviewed periodically by emergency care physicians for clarity and completeness. These forms may be on paper, although digital formats are preferred.

Limitations of EIFs include that parents must be able to have these forms available, either in hard copy or digitally, and they must be updated regularly in order to be effective. The best use of digital EIFs is those with a central repository, so they may be accessible to all providers irrespective of the type of electronic medical record used by their institution. However, there are significant barriers as ready access to this information is at odds with the principles of maintaining confidentiality of protected health information. Models for this do exist; Minnesota has implemented the Midwest Emergency Medical Services for Children Information System (**www.memscis.org**), which has "break-the-glass" functionality where information may be accessed in an emergency situation, bypassing traditional permissions for protected health information [12].

In order to provide the best care for these patients, a multilayered approach is important to prevent gaps in care. Most importantly, patients and families should be equipped with clear instructions on their or their child's care plan and an EIF for emergencies. Additionally, community providers should be prepared to initiate a workup and stabilize these patients when specialized resources are not immediately available. Lastly, subspecialists should partner with and be available to remotely support the patients, families, and community providers when questions arise in order to bring cohesion to an otherwise fragmented system.

References

1. Cohen E, Kuo DZ, Agrawal R, et al. Children with medical complexity: an emerging population for clinical and research initiatives. Pediatrics. 2011;127(3):529–38.
2. Turner A, Ricketts T, Leslie LK. Comparison of number and geographic distribution of pediatric subspecialists and patient proximity to specialized care in the US between 2003 and 2019. JAMA Pediatr. 2020;174(9):852–60.
3. Kamzan A, Jun-Ihn E, Kulkarni D. On the front lines of pediatric complex care: are we preparing emergency medicine residents? Hosp Pediatr. 2020;10(8):712–4. https://doi.org/10.1542/hpeds.2020-0141. Epub 2020 Jul 17
4. Hudgins JD, Monuteaux MC, Bourgeois FT, et al. Complexity and severity of pediatric patients treated at United States emergency departments. J Pediatr. 2017;186:145–149.e1.
5. Pulcini CD, Belardo Z, Ketterer T, Zorc JJ, Mollen CJ. Improving emergency care for children with medical complexity: parent and physicians' perspectives. Acad Pediatr. 2021;21(3):513–20. https://doi.org/10.1016/j.acap.2020.09.006.
6. Kuo DZ, Melguizo-Castro M, Goudie A, et al. Variation in child health care utilization by medical complexity. Matern Child Health J. 2015;19:40–8.
7. Bayer ND, Wang H, Yu JA, Kuo DZ, Halterman JS, Li Y. A national mental health profile of parents of children with medical complexity. Pediatrics. 2021;148(1):e2020023358. https://doi.org/10.1542/peds.2020-023358.
8. Lee LK, Mulvaney-Day N, Berger AM, Bhaumik U, Nguyen HT, Ward VL. The patient passport program: an intervention to improve patient-provider communication for hospitalized minority children and their families. Acad Pediatr. 2016;16(5):460–7. https://doi.org/10.1016/j.acap.2015.12.008. Epub 2015 Dec 23.
9. Copper TC, Jeffe DB, Ahmad FA, Abraham G, Yu F, Hickey B, Schnadower D. Emergency information forms for children with medical complexity: a qualitative study. Pediatr Emerg Care. 2020;36(6):e318–23. https://doi.org/10.1097/PEC.0000000000001443.

10. American College of Emergency Physicians. Emergency information form for children with special health care needs. Ann Emerg Med. 2010;56(3):315–6. https://doi.org/10.1016/j.annemergmed.2010.06.547.
11. American Academy of Pediatrics; Committee on Pediatric Emergency Medicine and Council on Clinical Information Technology; American College of Emergency Physicians; Pediatric Emergency Medicine Committee. Policy statement—emergency information forms and emergency preparedness for children with special health care needs. Pediatrics. 2010;125(4):829–37. https://doi.org/10.1542/peds.2010-0186. Epub 2010 Mar 29.
12. Pyles LA, Hines C, Patock M, Schied M, Chase J, Jamrozek K, Schiff JS. Development of a web-based database to manage American College of Emergency Physicians/American Academy of Pediatrics Emergency Information Forms. Acad Emerg Med. 2005;12(3):257–61.

Vomiting in a Child with a Metabolic Disorder

Margaret Nguyen, Youngeun Park, and Yue Huang

1 Case

A 10-year-old male with ornithine transcarbamylase deficiency, developmental delay, and gastrostomy tube presents with vomiting and altered mental status. He started having non-bilious, non-bloody vomiting yesterday, with more episodes today. His mother had started him on his "sick-day" plan of feeds by reducing protein in his diet and tried to keep him hydrated via his G-tube, but he continued to have emesis. His mother also noticed that he has been tired and wants to sleep during most of the day. In general, he has been taking his medications as prescribed and following his protein-restricted diet, but he stayed with a relative this past weekend who is less familiar with his diet. He has not had any fever, rhinorrhea, cough, diarrhea, or new rashes, though there was another sick child who had vomiting and diarrhea at school. His mother brought his emergency department letter from his pediatric genetic and metabolic specialist.

In the emergency department, he has temperature of 37.2 °C, heart rate of 128 beats/min, blood pressure of 109/65 mmHg, respiratory rate of 38 breaths/min, and oxygen saturation of 98% on room air. On exam, he is lethargic and difficult to awaken. His mucous membranes appear dry. He is tachycardic and tachypneic with mild subcostal retractions and clear breath sounds bilaterally. His abdomen is nontender with a G-tube in the left upper quadrant.

M. Nguyen (✉)
Department of Pediatrics, UCSF, San Francisco, CA, USA
e-mail: margaret.nguyen@ucsf.edu

Y. Park · Y. Huang
Department of Pediatrics, UCLA, Los Angeles, CA, USA
e-mail: ympark@mednet.ucla.edu; yuehuang@mednet.ucla.edu

A. Kamzan et al. (eds.), *Children with Medical Complexity in the Emergency Department*, https://doi.org/10.1007/978-3-031-62517-6_2

His initial labs are significant for the following:

- Complete blood count: white blood cell 12 × 10^3/mm^3, hemoglobin 13 g/dL, hematocrit 40%, platelet 352 × 10^3/mm^3, neutrophils 62%, lymphocytes 20%, monocytes 8%, eosinophils 1%, basophils 0.5%.
- Complete metabolic panel: sodium 140 mEq/L, potassium 3.1 mEq/L, chloride 105 mEq/L, carbon dioxide 22 mEq/L, blood urea nitrogen 18 mg/dL, creatinine 1.5 mg/dL, glucose 55 mg/dL, calcium 9.2 mg/dL, alanine transaminase 144 U/L, aspartate aminotransferase 115 U/L, total bilirubin 4.2 mg/dL, direct bilirubin 0.3 mg/dL, plasma ammonia 380 mcg/dL.
- Urinalysis: specific gravity 1.022, glucose negative, ketones trace, blood negative, protein negative, nitrites negative.
- Venous blood gas: pH 7.49, pCO_2 32 mmHg, bicarbonate 20 mEq/L, base excess −2.9 mmol/L, lactate 7 mg/dl.
- C-reactive protein 0.3 mg/L, procalcitonin 0.05 ng/mL.
- Blood and urine cultures pending.

2 Discussion Questions

1. What is the patient's diagnosis, and what evidence supports this?
2. What are the next steps in the management of this patient?
3. What complications should be anticipated?

3 Case Answers

1. The patient presents with tachypnea, dehydration, altered mental status, and hyperammonemia without metabolic acidosis in the setting of known urea cycle disorder (UCD), indicating that he is in metabolic crisis. The altered mental status is due to hyperammonemia.
2. Ensure that all protein intake is discontinued. Given the patient's hypoglycemia, an IV dextrose bolus should be administered immediately followed by D10 NS or D10 1/2 NS with electrolytes (as appropriate) at a rate of 1.5 times maintenance.
3. If the ammonia level continues to trend higher and above 500 mcg/dL, the patient may require hemodialysis. If there are provoked seizures, then antiepileptic medications may be needed. Fluid overload and cerebral edema may occur if all fluids and calories are given intravenously for a prolonged time.

4 Learning Objectives

1. Understand the major pathophysiologic principles of metabolic crisis.
2. Understand the initial management of metabolic crises.
3. Describe the complications that can occur with metabolic crises.

5 Discussion

5.1 *Inborn Errors of Metabolism and Metabolic Crisis*

Inborn errors of metabolism (IEMs) are genetic disorders that cause disruption of a metabolic pathway leading to either the accumulation of a toxic substrate proximal to the metabolic block, a deficiency of a product distal to the block, or a diversion of the substrate to an alternative pathway [1]. There are over 750 described IEMs [2] that can be categorized by the metabolites they primarily involve: protein—organic acidurias, aminoacidopathies, and urea cycle disorders; fats—fatty acid oxidation disorders; carbohydrates—glycogen storage diseases and galactosemia; and lysosomal storage diseases [3]. While IEMs individually are rare, the collective incidence is 1 in 800 births to 1 in 2500 births [4, 5].

Acute decompensation or metabolic crisis occurs when there is an accumulation of toxic metabolites or insufficient substrate for a patient's given energy needs. The typical triggers are conditions that physiologically challenge and increase catabolism such as acute infection, surgery, trauma, or fasting [6]. Metabolic crises can also be due to missed medication doses or nonadherence to dietary restrictions [6, 7], such as increased consumption of protein in UCD.

5.2 *Clinical Presentation*

Patients may present in crisis with nonspecific symptoms or in ways specific to their metabolic disease. Symptoms that overlap with other illnesses include lethargy, altered mental status, jitteriness, vomiting, dehydration, seizures, coma, and death [6, 8, 9]. Patients may also have symptoms that suggest an IEM, such as metabolic acidosis or hyperammonemia, which may lead to hyperpnea or tachypnea [10].

An undiagnosed patient can present with mild signs of disease or be in crisis. The patient may be a previously healthy child with rapid decompensation, organ injury, or developmental or global delay, all without a clear etiology [6]. For these patients, keep a broad differential, including sepsis, non-accidental trauma, toxic ingestion, congenital heart disease, endocrine emergencies (e.g., adrenal insufficiency), and other causes for children to present in extremis [6]. Though the Newborn Screen program is meant to help identify many congenital conditions shortly after delivery, including IEMs, a negative result is not always reliable. Not all IEMs are on the screen, and not every state tests for the same conditions. Additionally, the timing of when patients initially present can vary. Some have symptoms during the newborn period, while others have symptoms a few weeks into life, or potentially years later depending on the IEM and penetrance of the genetic condition [8, 11].

Based on the type of IEM, diagnosed patients can present in metabolic crisis with a variety of metabolic derangements (hypoglycemia, metabolic acidosis, hyperammonemia, ketoacidosis, lactic acidemia), hepatopathy, rhabdomyolysis, pancreatitis, or renal tubulopathy [6]. Patients and their families will likely have attempted to follow a sick-day regimen specific to their IEM that is created by a metabolic dietitian. For example, patients with UCD or propionic acidemia may be given formula or feeds free of protein for 24–48 h in an attempt to stop catabolism [10]. Caregivers will also monitor urine ketones, vomiting, and mental status and be in close communication with their subspecialty team. If the patient does not sufficiently improve at home, then they will be advised to seek care in an emergency department (ED).

5.3 Initial Evaluation and Management

When a patient with known IEM arrives in the ED, they typically present with an emergency letter, detailing the initial workup and management (Fig. 1). Labs should be collected prior to medical interventions that may obscure underlying pathophysiologic processes. These labs often include a metabolic derangement (complete metabolic panel, magnesium, phosphate, ammonia, blood gas, lactate, urinalysis) and basic infectious (complete blood count with differential, blood culture, urine culture) evaluation [8, 12]. The results of the workup will vary depending on the type of IEM. Of note, serum ammonia levels must be obtained without a tourniquet, from free-flowing blood, and sent STAT on ice to yield accurate results. If there is concern for an IEM in an undiagnosed patient, sending plasma amino acids, urine organic acids, plasma acylcarnitine profile, free and total carnitine, and carnitine esters in addition to basic labs may help reveal the diagnosis [8].

Immediate therapy of acute encephalopathy due to IEM involves measures to decrease the production of offending metabolites and increase their excretion [2]. Therefore, adequate hydration and good urine output are imperative because many metabolites are freely filtered at the glomerulus [2]. High calories without protein should be administered immediately via IV D10 ½ NS or D10 NS with electrolytes (as appropriate) at 1.5 times maintenance to reverse or avoid catabolism. If D10 is unavailable, then consider starting D5 until D10 is available. For hypoglycemia, administer a D10 bolus prior to starting maintenance IV fluids. In a patient with severe acidosis, a bicarbonate infusion can partially correct the acidosis; however, bicarbonate should be used with caution since it can cause hypernatremia, cerebral edema, or cerebral hemorrhage [2].

Disease-specific therapy should be initiated with the guidance of a genetic and metabolic specialist (Table 1). For patients with UCDs like the one presented in this case, specialized treatments may be given to divert a toxic substrate to a benign excretable form. Oral forms of ammonia lowering agents can be given if the patient is tolerating oral intake after initial stabilization and include glycerol phenylbutyrate PO, sodium phenylbutyrate PO, and sodium benzoate PO (which has off-label use in the United States). If the patient requires intravenous nitrogen scavengers, sodium phenylacetate/sodium benzoate IV infusion can be used but requires central line access. Substrates that replenish the urea cycle are also given including citrulline PO or arginine IV (depending on oral tolerance). In particular, arginine hydrochloride (acidic) can help patients with alkalosis. If ammonia levels are very high,

Diagnosis: Ornithine Transcarbamylase Deficiency (OTC)

OTC is an inherited disorder of the urea cycle. Patients with OTC can have episodic metabolic crises with hyperammonemia, triggered by fasting, vomiting or intercurrent illness. If not treated, these episodes may result in permanent brain injury, coma, or even death. Although OTC deficiency is X-linked, females with partial OTC may have symptoms and affected females need to be treated with the same care as male patients.

Attention Triage Nurse and Emergency room personnel:
This patient should be assessed ON ARRIVAL to the Emergency Department, even if he or she looks well. Delays could result in sudden death.

EMERGENCY-ROOM MANAGEMENT IN ACUTE ILLNESS:

1. Immediately start IV glucose D10 ½ NS or D10 NS with electrolytes (as appropriate) at 1.5 times maintenance with a max rate of 150 ml/hr (if hypoglycemic the patient may need a D10 bolus). If D10 is not available, start D5 until the D10 is available. This will stop the protein breakdown of the patient's own body.
2. Labs: STAT ammonia (on ice, transport STAT to lab, free-flowing blood with no tourniquet). Other labs to consider: glucose, electrolytes, liver function studies, CBC with differential, urinalysis for ketones/specific gravity, blood and urine cultures (if indicated).
3. DO NOT administer TPN or protein unless specifically discussed with the geneticist.
4. Call the page operator at (800) 800-8000 and ask to speak with the Genetics and Metabolic Specialist on call.
5. Other specialized treatments such as arginine and ammonia lowering agents may be given after discussion with the geneticist. If the ammonia is very high, hemodialysis may be considered.

Fig. 1 Sample emergency department letter. Patients with a diagnosed IEM and their caregivers often present to the emergency department when in metabolic crisis and will have a letter explaining the initial evaluation and management for the patient's particular disease

Table 1 Management strategies for IEMs after discussion with the genetic and metabolic specialist

Inborn error of metabolism	Examples of treatment options
Organic aciduria	Levocarnitine N-carbamylglutamate Dietary management specific to the IEM
Amino acidopathies	Intralipids Cofactor supplementation (e.g., vitamin B6) Ammonia scavengers Dietary management specific to the IEM Orthotopic liver transplant
Urea cycle defect	Ammonia scavengers (e.g., sodium benzoate, sodium phenylbutyrate) N-carbamylglutamate Arginine or citrulline Dialysis
Fatty acid oxidation disorders	Intralipids are contraindicated MCT oil (VLCAD)
Glycogen storage diseases	Raw cornstarch
Lysosomal storage diseases	Enzyme replacement Hematopoietic stem cell transplant

hemodialysis may be necessary. In other IEMs, intralipids may be needed to supplement calories to prevent further catabolism, and cofactors such as vitamin B6 or B12 can be administered to improve the function of a defective enzyme [2].

5.4 Complications and Comorbidities

The complications related to metabolic crises can range from correctable issues such as electrolyte abnormalities to more serious ones, such as cerebral edema and death. Any patient with an IEM who is presenting with altered mental status can be at risk of being unable to protect their airway and respiratory failure. Over the long term, repeated metabolic crises can also cause neurological sequelae that affect development or lead to multi-organ damage, including renal or hepatic insufficiency or failure. Please see Table 2 for examples of complications and comorbidities that patients with IEM may develop.

Patients who have an IEM may also have other ongoing medical needs. Those with developmental delay may have difficulty expressing their symptoms, and their neurological exam may be challenging. Though not a complication from metabolic crises or IEMs, patients may have a gastrostomy tube to ensure consistent specialized medical formula feeds. For some patients, morbidity comes from the treatment

Table 2 Complications and comorbidities of IEMs

Inborn error of metabolism[a]	Examples of complications and comorbidities
Protein related disorders: organic acidurias, aminoacidopathies, and urea cycle disorders	Maple syrup urine disease: neurotoxic levels of leucine lead to seizure, hallucinations, lethargy, and vomiting and can result in cerebral edema, coma, and death [8] Methylmalonic acidemia: metabolic acidosis, metabolic stroke, pancreatitis, chronic kidney disease, growth faltering, regression, developmental delay [8, 9, 14] Urea cycle diseases: hyperammonemia, cerebral edema, global developmental delay, intellectual disability, and spasticity [8]
Fatty acid oxidation disorders: acyl CoA deficiencies, carnitine palmitoyltransferase deficiencies	Fatty acid oxidation disorders: hypoketotic hypoglycemia (leading to seizures and encephalopathy [8]), cardiomyopathy, arrhythmia [2, 11], hypotonia, retinopathy, hepatic dysfunction [13]
Carbohydrate related disorders: glycogen storage diseases and galactosemia	Pompe disease: hypertrophic cardiomyopathy, arrhythmia [2, 11], hepatomegaly, hypotonia, respiratory failure [15][b] von Gierke disease: lactic acidosis, hypertriglyceridemia, elevated transaminases, renal failure [3, 16] Galactosemia: failure to thrive, speech delay, hepatic failure, cataracts, premature ovarian failure, *E. coli* sepsis [3]

[a]Lysosomal storage disorders do not typically present with metabolic crisis and so are not included in these examples

[b]Pompe disease is a glycogen storage and lysosomal storage disease [15]

of the disease. For example, patients with methylmalonic acidemia can have a renal transplant, and patients with mucopolysaccharidoses I and II may have a history of a stem cell transplant [3]. Though these patients are less likely to have a metabolic crisis since their transplants should help alleviate their disease, ED teams may also need to consider illness due to or affecting the patient's transplanted organ when they present.

Sick patients with an IEM require careful evaluation and a high suspicion for an ongoing metabolic crisis. Due to the complexity and rarity of their condition, the patients' caregivers and genetic and metabolic subspecialty teams are essential resources to their care. When they are showing signs of metabolic crisis, rapid decompensation and significant complications can occur; therefore, early intervention and frequent re-evaluations are cornerstones of management.

6 Review Questions

1. A 5-year-old male patient with very-long-chain acyl-CoA dehydrogenase deficiency with frequent ear infections presents with emesis and dyspnea after surgery for tympanostomy and myringotomy tube placement. He appears tired and is tachypneic. In addition to checking a CBC, point-of-care glucose, CMP, magnesium, phosphate, creatinine kinase, blood gas, and urinalysis, what other examination should be done at this time?

    (A) Retinal eye exam
    (B) Echocardiogram and electrocardiogram
    (C) Abdominal ultrasound
    (D) Muscle biopsy

2. A 3-year-old male with maple syrup urine disease presents with fever, altered mental status, and emesis. He also has rhinorrhea and a cough that started two days ago and has decreased intake of his specialized formula. He is tachycardic with a heart rate of 138 beats/min, has dry mucous membranes, and had two wet diapers in the last 24 h. The ED medical team reviewed his emergency department letter and has initiated the appropriate evaluation. He was given two 20 ml/kg normal saline boluses with improvement in his heart rate to 106 beats/min. He was also started D10 ½ NS running at 1.5 times maintenance and has been waiting for more than 24 h for transfer to an institution with a pediatric genetic and metabolic subspecialist. While waiting, he becomes sleepier and then obtunded. What could explain his change in mental status?

    (A) Worsening hyperammonemia
    (B) Fluid overload and cerebral edema
    (C) Meningitis or encephalitis due to CNS infection
    (D) Intracranial hemorrhage

3. A 7-year-old male with propionic acidemia presents to the ED with cough, vomiting, and lethargy. On physical examination, he is lethargic but arousable. The vital signs showed mild tachycardia but are otherwise unremarkable. The initial labs reveal the following: sodium 132 mEq/L, potassium 3.5 mEq/L, bicarbonate 11 mEq/L, blood urea nitrogen 20 mg/dL, creatinine 1.2 mg/dL, glucose 35 mg/dL, and ammonia 348 mcg/dL. The patient was made NPO and was given a D10 bolus. What is the next best step?

   (A) D10NS at 1.5 times maintenance
   (B) D10NS at maintenance since he already received a bolus
   (C) IV sodium phenylacetate/sodium benzoate
   (D) IV sodium bicarbonate

7 Answers

1. **B.** Echocardiogram and electrocardiogram. Patients with very-long-chain acyl-CoA dehydrogenase deficiency are at risk of developing cardiac related complications. The disorder causes accumulation of fatty acids in the cytoplasm and lysosomes of cardiac tissue and misalignment of cardiac myofibrils. This leads to inflammation and inefficient contractions that cause hypertrophic cardiomyopathy [13]. The patient is presenting with vomiting after undergoing surgery, which is physiologically stressful and may have triggered a crisis episode. In addition to the usual evaluation for possible infection and checking electrolytes, this patient is experiencing dyspnea and should also be evaluated for congestive heart failure and for arrhythmias. Patients with fatty acid oxidation disorders can also develop retinopathy, hepatopathy, skeletal myopathy, and neurological sequelae due to the inability to utilize different types of fatty acids; however, the evaluation for these is not as urgent.
2. **B.** Fluid overload and cerebral edema. The patient has been fluid resuscitated with normal saline boluses to support his hydration and cardiovascular status. Transfer to tertiary or quaternary care centers can take many hours depending on where the closest center is located. Though initially stabilized, the patient needs re-evaluation and potentially changes in how calories are provided. The safest way to provide calories is through enteral feeds; however, that is not always feasible initially. After stabilizing the patient, a plan should be made with the subspecialist on the next steps in management. Though patients with MSUD can experience hyperammonemia, the levels are not as severe as in urea cycle disorders, and this patient was already stabilized with dextrose-containing fluids that should stop catabolizing processes. It is possible for the patient to have a CNS infection, with his symptoms of fever, emesis, and altered mental status; however, it is less likely given his overall picture. A spontaneous intracranial bleed is also less likely.
3. **Answer A.** D10NS at 1.5 times maintenance. The primary goals of emergency care in a patient in metabolic crisis include correction of hypoglycemia, suppres-

sion of catabolism, suppression of toxic metabolite formation, correction of metabolic acidosis, and correction of hyperammonemia (usually in urea cycle disorders). The patient received a D10 bolus to correct his hypoglycemia. The most important and best next step would be to start D10NS at a higher than maintenance rate to provide enough calories and reverse catabolism. Sodium phenylacetate/sodium benzoate IV is an ammonia scavenger that can be used for hyperammonemia, but should be discussed with the genetic and metabolic subspecialist first. Bicarbonate can be administered to counter acidosis though it should not precede the initiation of maintenance fluids.

8 Takeaway Points

1. Patients with a diagnosed IEM will often have an emergency department letter that explains what initial evaluation and management should be completed.
2. Depending on the IEM, monitor for electrolyte abnormalities and multi-organ system injury.
3. The complications of IEM can be insidious and be confused with symptoms of other illnesses, such as infection, dehydration, or intracranial processes (increased intracranial pressure, intracranial hemorrhage, non-accidental trauma).
4. Parents often know whether their children are close to their baseline or whether previous crises have resulted in similar episodes of altered mental status. Use their breadth of knowledge to better evaluate the child.

References

1. Ferreira CR, van Karnebeek CDM, Vockley J, et al. A proposed nosology of inborn errors of metabolism. Genet Med. 2019;21:102–6. https://doi.org/10.1038/s41436-018-0022-8.
2. Saudubray JM, Garcia-Cazorla A. Inborn errors of metabolism overview: pathophysiology, manifestations, evaluation, and management. Pediatr Clin N Am. 2018;65(2):179–208. https://doi.org/10.1016/j.pcl.2017.11.002.
3. Vergano SAS. Inborn errors of metabolism: becoming ready for rare. Pediatr Rev. 2022;43(7):371–83. https://doi.org/10.1542/pir.2022-005088.
4. Applegarth DA, Toone JR, Lowry RB. Incidence of inborn errors of metabolism in British Columbia, 1969–1996. Pediatrics. 2000;105(1):e10. https://doi.org/10.1542/peds.105.1.e10.
5. Sanderson S, Green A, Preece MA, Burton H. The incidence of inherited metabolic disorders in the West Midlands, UK. Arch Dis Child. 2006;91(11):896–9. https://doi.org/10.1136/adc.2005.091637.
6. Strauss KA. Metabolic crisis. In: Lucking SE, Maffei FA, editors. Pediatric critical care: text and study guide. 2nd ed. Springer: Cham; 2022. p. 1351–96. https://doi.org/10.1007/978-3-030-53363-2_44.
7. Baumgartner MR, Horster F, Dionisi-Vici C, et al. Proposed guidelines for the diagnosis and management of methylmalonic and propionic acidemia. Orphanet J Rare Dis. 2014;9:130. https://doi.org/10.1186/s13023-014-0130-8.

8. Rice GM, Steiner RD. Inborn errors of metabolism (metabolic disorders). Pediatr Rev. 2016;37(1):3–17. https://doi.org/10.1542/pir.2014-0122.
9. Ewing PH, Wiebe RA. Evidence-based management of metabolic emergencies in the pediatric emergency department. Pediatr Emerg Med Pract. 2009;6(10):1–16.
10. Claudius I, Fluharty C, Boles R. The emergency department approach to newborn and childhood metabolic crisis. Emerg Med Clin North Am. 2005;23(3):843–83. https://doi.org/10.1016/j.emc.2005.03.010.
11. Agana M, Frueh J, Kamboj M, et al. Common metabolic disorder (inborn errors of metabolism) concerns in primary care practice. Ann Transl Med. 2018;6(24):469. https://doi.org/10.21037/atm.2018.12.34.
12. Lindor NM, Karnes PS. Initial assessment of infants and children with suspected inborn errors of metabolism. Mayo Clin Proc. 1995;70(10):987–8. https://doi.org/10.4065/70.10.987.
13. Merritt JL, MacLeod E, Jurecka A, et al. Clinical manifestations and management of fatty acid oxidation disorders. Rev Endocr Metab Disord. 2020;21(4):479–93. https://doi.org/10.1007/s11154-020-09568-3.
14. Horster F, Baumgartner MR, Viardot C, et al. Long-term outcome in methylmalonic acidurias is influenced by the underlying defect (mut^0, mut^-, cblA, cblB). Pediatr Res. 2007;62(2):225–30. https://doi.org/10.1203/PDR.0b013e3180a0325f.
15. Kishnani P, Steiner RD, Bali D, et al. Pompe disease diagnosis and management guideline. Genet Med. 2006;8:267–88. https://doi.org/10.1097/01.gim.0000218152.87434.f3.
16. Oster Y, Wexler ID, Heyman SN, et al. Recoverable, record-high lactic acidosis in a patient with glycogen storage disease type 1: a mixed type A and type B lactate disorder. Case Rep Med. 2016;2016:4362743. https://doi.org/10.1155/2016/4362743.

Further Reading

Strauss KA. Metabolic crisis. In: Lucking SE, Maffei FA, editors. Pediatric critical care: text and study guide. 2nd ed. Springer: Cham; 2022. p. 1351–96. https://doi.org/10.1007/978-3-030-53363-2_44.

Vergano SAS. Inborn errors of metabolism: becoming ready for rare. Pediatr Rev. 2022;43(7):371–83. https://doi.org/10.1542/pir.2022-005088.

A Patient with Leukemia and a Fever

Rabia Cheema, Miriam Beyder, and Camille Hamilton

1 Case

A 5-year-old female with a past medical history of acute lymphoid leukemia presents to the emergency department with fever. She was discharged from the hospital 8 days ago after completing induction chemotherapy. Her mother reports that for the past 2 days, she has appeared fatigued and has been sleeping more than usual. She has also been complaining of abdominal pain and has had several episodes of non-bloody, non-bilious emesis starting earlier today. She reports that she does not have any dysuria or diarrhea. She does not have any respiratory symptoms, including cough and congestion. There are no known sick contacts. In terms of medications, she has been receiving ondansetron as needed for nausea and emesis, docusate as needed for constipation, and trimethoprim-sulfamethoxazole for prophylaxis against opportunistic infections on Saturdays and Sundays.

Upon examination, vitals are notable for a temperature of 39.4 °C, a heart rate of 145 beats/min, and a respiratory rate of 20 breaths/min. Her blood pressure is 100/72 mmHg, and her oxygen saturation is 96% on room air. She is alert but appears tired. Her central venous catheter site appears clean without overlying skin changes. Her lungs are clear to auscultation bilaterally, and cardiovascular exam is remarkable for tachycardia with regular rhythm. Her abdominal examination is notable for exquisite tenderness to palpation in the right lower quadrant with rebound and guarding. Laboratory testing is performed. Her complete blood count is notable for a white blood count of 0.76/μL, with an absolute neutrophil count of 340/μL, hemoglobin of 9.1 g/dL, and platelet count of 53,000/μL.

R. Cheema (✉) · M. Beyder · C. Hamilton
David Geffen School of Medicine, UCLA, Los Angeles, CA, USA
e-mail: rcheema@mednet.ucla.edu; mbeyder@mednet.ucla.edu; camillehamilton@mednet.ucla.edu

A. Kamzan et al. (eds.), *Children with Medical Complexity in the Emergency Department*, https://doi.org/10.1007/978-3-031-62517-6_3

2 Discussion Questions

1. What are the next best steps in management?
2. What additional workup would you consider in this case?

3 Case Answers

1. This patient is presenting with fever in the setting of neutropenia induced by recent completion of induction chemotherapy for acute lymphoid leukemia. The next best steps in management are to obtain blood cultures from all lumens of her central venous catheter site as well as peripheral blood if possible and immediate initiation of empiric broad-spectrum antibiotic therapy with an antipseudomonal beta-lactam, a fourth-generation cephalosporin, or a carbapenem [1].
2. While the patient denies dysuria, cultures from urine should be obtained using a clean-catch technique. With this patient's presentation, a diagnosis of neutropenic enterocolitis, also known as typhlitis, must also be evaluated with computed tomography or magnetic resonance imaging.

4 Learning Objectives

1. Define neutropenic fever, and create a differential diagnosis, including infectious and noninfectious etiologies.
2. Understand the initial management of neutropenic fever, including risk stratification of patients, common pathogens to consider, and empiric antimicrobial therapy.
3. Discuss the etiology and management of non-chemotherapy-induced neutropenia in the pediatric population.

5 Discussion

Pediatric patients with cancer make up a significant portion of the population of children with medical complexity. Fever in the pediatric cancer patient who is undergoing myelosuppressive chemotherapy or has received a hematopoietic stem cell transplant is a common reason for presentation to the emergency department and should be considered an oncological emergency. Prompt evaluation and treatment are critical as these children are at increased risk for developing life-threatening infections, with a recent meta-analysis estimating a mortality rate of 3%. In the same studies, an etiology was identified in only 20% of patients; of those, about 90% were found to have bacterial infections [2].

For this patient population, fever is defined by the Infectious Diseases Society of America as a single temperature greater than or equal to 38.3 °C or two measurements of 38.0–38.2 °C within 1 h. Neutropenia is defined as an absolute neutrophil count less than 1500 cells/microL. It can be further classified by severity: mild, with an absolute neutrophil count of 1000–1500 cells/μL; moderate, with an absolute neutrophil count of 500–1000 cells/μL; and severe, with an absolute neutrophil count less than 500 cells/μL. For patients who have undergone chemotherapy, the nadir of neutropenia (alongside anemia and thrombocytopenia) usually occurs in the 7–10 days following treatment. It is estimated that over a third of these patients may demonstrate febrile episodes during this neutropenic period prior to bone marrow recovery [3].

As mentioned, infection is a leading cause of fever in a patient with chemotherapy-induced neutropenia and should be at the forefront of a provider's differential diagnosis and management. The risk of serious bacterial infection increases with decreasing absolute neutrophil count. The majority of these patients are not identified to have bacteremia, as the etiology is presumed to be transient gut translocation secondary to mucosal breakdown, which is often not detected with a blood culture. However, the morbidity and mortality associated with serious bacterial infections in this population warrant aggressive treatment with hospitalization for parenteral antibiotic therapy and close monitoring until they demonstrate both resolution of fever and evidence of bone marrow recovery.

These patients are also at risk for other infectious causes of neutropenic fever, including viral and fungal infections. Most common are respiratory viruses, but herpes simplex and varicella zoster are also relatively prevalent. Of note, hematopoietic stem cell transplant patients are at particular risk for certain viral infections, of which Epstein-Barr virus, cytomegalovirus, and human herpesvirus 6 are the most common. Additionally, certain patients who are considered high risk as noted below are more predisposed to fungal infections [1].

While infectious causes should always be the first consideration in these patients, other causes for chemotherapy-induced neutropenic fever may be considered if initial workup is unremarkable. Often, the fever may be related to the cancer in and of itself. Similarly, the fever may ultimately be attributed to supportive management of the cancer, related to either a drug reaction or a transfusion reaction. Additionally, many oncologic patients are at high risk for venous thromboembolism, and fever can be a presenting sign. Finally, patients with evidence of oncologic disease in the central nervous system may experience dysautonomia and present with febrile episodes in addition to other vital sign abnormalities.

Any patient with febrile neutropenia that is ill-appearing, has concern for dangerous underlying etiology, or has a high-risk oncologic diagnosis or stem cell transplant should be admitted with prompt administration of antibiotics. Patients with high-risk oncologic disease include those with acute myeloid leukemia (AML), patients with high-risk or relapsed acute lymphoid leukemia (ALL), patients receiving high-dose steroids, patients with known prolonged neutropenia, and patients with stem cell transplant without T-cell reconstitution or those receiving treatment for graft-versus-host disease (GvHD) [1]. Ideally, antibiotic administration should be initiated within 1 h of triage [1] and should not be delayed for laboratory workup or imaging. As noted, workup should include blood cultures from all lumens of any central venous catheters, a peripheral culture if possible, laboratory evaluation including a complete blood count with differential and electrolyte panel, and a urinalysis with urine culture if a midstream clean catch can be reasonably obtained. Evaluation should be mindful of neutropenic precautions, notably no rectal temperatures or rectal delivery of medications, and no bladder catheterization to avoid possible introduction of bacteria. Imaging should be tailored to a patient's symptoms [1], such as a chest radiograph or respiratory viral testing in the setting of respiratory symptoms.

Of particular note is abdominal imaging, such as with computed tomography, in patients with complaints of severe abdominal pain or tenderness as neutropenic enterocolitis, or typhlitis, is a life-threatening complication that must be considered. Neutropenic patients are at particular risk for this complication due to increased gut translocation of enteric pathogens. For those patients in whom typhlitis is suspected, the approach includes both medical and surgical management. At a minimum, these patients should be placed on bowel rest with broadening of antimicrobial coverage to include anaerobic coverage. Prompt surgical consultation should be obtained, and the need for surgical intervention should be frequently reassessed. Patients with signs of hemodynamic instability, clinical deterioration, perforation, or bleeding are likely to require emergent surgical management. Finally, while typhlitis is necessary to consider with this presentation, it is important to recall that these patients are still at risk for other common but serious causes of abdominal pain such as appendicitis and cholecystitis.

In high-risk patients, fungal infection should also be considered in cases of prolonged febrile neutropenia, defined as greater than or equal to 96 h. Empiric antifungal therapy is no longer routinely recommended in patients other than those with stem cell transplants. Furthermore, labs to evaluate for fungal infection are not routinely recommended, but imaging of the chest, abdomen, and sinuses may be considered [1].

Antibiotic choice is generally an antipseudomonal beta-lactam, a fourth-generation cephalosporin, or a carbapenem [1] (Table 1). In a clinically unstable patient, a second anti-gram-negative agent or glycopeptide (typically vancomycin) should be considered [1]. Vancomycin should also be initiated in patients with any known hardware, especially in the setting of recent orthopedic intervention, or known MRSA colonization. Patients will require hospitalization with empiric antibiotic coverage until they are afebrile for greater than 24 h and showing signs of bone marrow recovery [1]. For oncologic patients who do not meet high-risk criteria as described above, outpatient management with oral antibiotic administration and close follow-up and monitoring can be considered in discussion with the patient's pediatric oncology team [1]. We would recommend against outpatient management without oncology consultation, and it is always an appropriate option to admit these patients out of caution.

Otherwise healthy children who present with fever in the emergency department may have an incidental finding of neutropenia. Neutropenia is a common transient

Table 1 Antibiotic management of febrile neutropenia

Patient population	Clinical considerations:	Recommended antibiotic choice
Low-risk febrile neutropenia	Low risk as defined by not meeting high-risk criteria, such as low-risk ALL and solid tumors without prolonged neutropenia	Can consider outpatient observation or oral antibacterial therapy such as levofloxacin or ciprofloxacin and amoxicillin/clavulanic acid in conversation with the patient's oncologist
High-risk febrile neutropenia	High-risk oncologic patients: AML, high-risk or relapsed ALL, high-dose steroids, known prolonged neutropenia, HSCT without T-cell reconstitution, or receiving treatment for GvHD	Antipseudomonal beta-lactam such as piperacillin-tazobactam, fourth-generation cephalosporin such as cefepime, or carbapenem such as meropenem as empiric monotherapy
Clinically unstable patients, initial therapy	Vital sign instability including fluid-refractory tachycardia and hypotension	Addition of a second anti-gram-negative agent or glycopeptide such as vancomycin to above monotherapy
Known hardware or MRSA colonization	Examples include patients with bone tumors with orthopedic implants or recent orthopedic intervention, patients with Ommaya reservoir or VP shunt. Ports alone not considered hardware requiring broadening to include glycopeptide use unless otherwise indicated	Addition of glycopeptide such as vancomycin to above monotherapy
Concern for typhlitis	Severe abdominal pain or bloody stools	Addition of anaerobic coverage such as metronidazole or clindamycin to above monotherapy
Clinically unstable patients, broadening if no improvement	See above for clinically unstable definition	Include coverage for resistant gram-negative, gram-positive, and anaerobic bacteria, a sample combination being meropenem and vancomycin
High-risk febrile neutropenia with prolonged fever and neutropenia (>96 h)	See above for high-risk patient definition	If patient with hematopoietic stem cell transplant, consider antifungal therapy such as fluconazole in discussion with infectious disease and primary oncologist

finding in immunocompetent children. The most likely etiology for these patients is postinfectious transient marrow suppression, with viruses being the most common pathogens [4]. In fact, otherwise healthy, well-appearing pediatric patients who present with the first episode of isolated neutropenia are at low risk for hematologic diagnoses or malignancy [5]. In these patients, there is usually full bone marrow recovery without any intervention. Nonetheless, close attention should be paid to a complete blood count showing multiple deranged cell lines, which could be concerning for a hematologic malignancy. Additional signs of malignancy can be assessed via a careful history including generalized symptoms such as chronic fatigue, weight loss, or night sweats suggestive of malignancy and physical examination looking for areas of tenderness or pain that could be suggestive of a solid tumor. Lab work can be obtained to assess electrolyte status and other signs of tumor lysis syndrome, including elevations in uric acid and lactate dehydrogenase. Additionally, a physical exam finding of hypersplenism can account for neutropenia due to splenic sequestration [6]. Another potential cause of non-chemotherapy neutropenia may be an adverse drug reaction, a generally benign etiology that resolves with removal of the offending agent [6]. A careful history of recent new drug exposure or medication changes, including antibiotics, anticonvulsants, and anti-inflammatory agents, can be an indication of drug-induced neutropenia [7]. Other etiologies, including immune disorders, bone marrow failure disorders, and congenital neutropenia syndromes, are far less common and indeed quite rare [7]. Many inherited syndromes will present with classic physical findings, including skeletal abnormalities, characteristic facies, or failure to thrive as well as recurrent infections requiring antibiotic treatment and notable family history (Table 2).

There is a lack of guidance and consensus on the management of febrile neutropenia in otherwise healthy children despite the risk of serious bacterial infection being significantly lower and in fact exceedingly rare as compared to children with

Table 2 Differential diagnosis of febrile neutropenia

Chemotherapy induced	Non-chemotherapy induced

Viral
• Respiratory virus
• Herpes simplex
• Varicella
• *If hematopoietic stem cell transplant:*
  • Epstein-Barr virus
  • Cytomegalovirus
  • Human herpesvirus 6
Bacterial
• Bacteremia/central line-associated bloodstream infection
• Gastrointestinal
• Respiratory
• Urinary
• Skin/soft tissue
Fungal
• Candida
• Aspergillus
Noninfectious
• Drug induced
• Cancer related
• Thromboembolism
• Transfusion reaction
• Dysautonomia from central nervous system disease
	Postinfectious
	Drug induced
	Immune disorder
	• Chronic idiopathic neutropenia
	• Autoimmune neutropenia
	Hypersplenism
	Bone marrow failure
	• Malnutrition
	• Aplastic anemia
	• Fanconi anemia
	• Diamond-Blackfan
	• Dyskeratosis congenita
	Congenital neutropenia
	• Kostmann syndrome
	• Cyclic neutropenia
	• Shwachman-Diamond syndrome
	• Chediak-Higashi syndrome
	Malignancy

a malignancy. Of note, the risk of infection in children with non-chemotherapy-induced neutropenia varies depending on the underlying cause [6]. Management of otherwise healthy children with neutropenia is often extrapolated from guidelines for chemotherapy-induced febrile neutropenia and can result in significant variation in the workup and management, including the need for hospitalization and antibiotic administration. However, recent studies have suggested that these patients may safely be managed without hospitalization or empiric antibiotics [8].

In summary, it is critical to understand that fever is a commonly noted complication in a patient who is neutropenic in the setting of myelosuppressive chemotherapy or a hematopoietic stem cell transplant, and this represents an oncological emergency with prompt need for evaluation and treatment. In contrast, fever in another otherwise healthy child with an incidental finding of neutropenia is likely to have a more benign outcome, but further research is needed to help create consensus and guidance for management.

6 Review Questions

1. A 12-year-old patient with high-risk acute lymphoblastic leukemia in induction therapy is sent to the emergency department from an oncology clinic for a temperature of 39 degree Celsius and an absolute neutrophil count of 160 cells/μL. She remains febrile in the ED where additional vitals include a heart rate of 110 beats/min, respiratory rate of 12 breaths/min, and blood pressure of 100/60 mmHg. Patient's physical exam is notable for mild rhinorrhea but is otherwise unremarkable. What is the appropriate management choice for this patient?

   (A) Discharge with cephalexin prescription and close follow-up
   (B) Admit and initiate monotherapy with cefepime
   (C) Admit and initiate antibiotic therapy with cefepime and vancomycin
   (D) Admit and initiate antibiotic therapy with cefepime, vancomycin, and caspofungin

2. An otherwise healthy 2-year-old patient presents to the emergency department with fever for 3 days. He is noted to have rhinorrhea, cough, and congestion. A rapid PCR is positive for respiratory syncytial virus. A complete blood count in the emergency department is only notable for an absolute neutrophil count of 750 cells/μL. Physical exam reveals a well-appearing child. He does not take any medications. No prior laboratory testing is available. What is the next best step in management?

   (A) Blood culture, urine culture, and empiric antibiotics
   (B) Admission for observation only with serial monitoring of labs
   (C) Outpatient observation with close follow-up with his primary care physician
   (D) Outpatient observation with close follow-up with a pediatric hematologist

3. A 2-year-old patient with acute myeloid leukemia presents to the emergency department for fever for 1 day. Labs are notable for an absolute neutrophil count of 150 cells/μL. Bacterial blood cultures are obtained from her port site, and empiric antibiotics are started. Parents endorse that she has been complaining of abdominal pain with multiple episodes of emesis and inability to tolerate oral intake. Which of the following next steps is most appropriate in terms of workup and management?

    (A) Obtain a catheterized urine specimen to evaluate for a urinary tract infection.
    (B) Proceed with computed tomography of the abdomen and pelvis, and consult pediatric surgery.
    (C) Administer rectal acetaminophen, given fever and emesis.
    (D) Obtain fungal blood cultures, and start empiric antifungals for high-risk neutropenia.

7 Answers

1. **B.** Admit and initiate monotherapy with cefepime. This patient has high-risk febrile neutropenia given her high-risk acute lymphoblastic leukemia diagnosis and needs to be admitted with prompt initiation of antibiotic therapy. Given that she is clinically stable without any known hardware or MRSA colonization, monotherapy with a fourth-generation cephalosporin antibiotic such as cefepime is sufficient as initial therapy. Empiric fungal therapy is not indicated.
2. **C**. Outpatient observation with close follow-up with his primary care physician. This patient is an otherwise healthy child who has been noted to have an incidental finding of moderate neutropenia in the setting of fever with a confirmed viral illness. He is well-appearing. Recent studies suggest that there is low likelihood of a hematologic diagnosis or malignancy. It is appropriate to monitor this patient in the outpatient setting with his primary care physician. Further testing, empiric antibiotics, admission to the hospital, or referral to hematology are not necessary at this time.
3. **B**. Proceed with computed tomography of the abdomen and pelvis, and consult pediatric surgery. Given the finding of abdominal pain in the setting of febrile neutropenia, a diagnosis of neutropenic enterocolitis, or typhlitis, must be considered, and abdominal imaging should be ordered. These patients may be considered for surgical management, and thus a surgical consult is also warranted. Consideration should be given to fungal etiology in cases of prolonged duration of febrile neutropenia in high-risk patients, which is defined as greater than or equal to 96 h. However, empiric antifungals are no longer routinely recommended. Additionally, it is important to maintain neutropenic precautions, which include avoiding rectal temperatures, rectal delivery of medications, or bladder catheterization.

8 Takeaway Points

1. The differential diagnosis of febrile neutropenia in patients undergoing chemotherapy includes both infectious and noninfectious causes.
2. Given the morbidity and mortality associated with serious bacterial infections, all children with chemotherapy-associated febrile neutropenia should be evaluated promptly.
3. High-risk patients should receive empiric antibiotics with an antipseudomonal beta-lactam, fourth-generation cephalosporin, or carbapenem and be hospitalized until resolution of fever and evidence of bone marrow recovery.
4. In a clinically unstable patient, a second anti-gram-negative agent or glycopeptide (typically vancomycin) should be considered. Vancomycin should also be initiated in patients with any known hardware, especially in the setting of recent orthopedic intervention or known MRSA colonization.
5. Abdominal imaging should be ordered in patients with complaints of severe abdominal pain or tenderness to evaluate for neutropenic enterocolitis, also known as typhlitis.
6. Special considerations for this patient population include neutropenic precautions, notably no rectal temperatures, rectal delivery of medications, or bladder catheterization to avoid possible introduction of bacteria.
7. Otherwise healthy children who present with a first episode of febrile neutropenia may be managed less conservatively and do not usually require hospitalization and empiric antibiotics.

References

1. Lehrnbecher T, Robinson PD, Ammann RA, Fisher B, Patel P, Phillips R, Beauchemin MP, Carlesse F, Castagnola E, Davis BL, Elgarten CW, Groll AH, Haeusler GM, Koenig C, Santolaya ME, Tissing WJE, Wolf J, Alexander S, Hu H, Dupuis LL, Sung L. Guideline for the management of fever and neutropenia in pediatric patients with cancer and hematopoietic cell transplantation recipients: 2023 update. J Clin Oncol. 2023;41(9):1774–85.
2. Boeriu E, et al. Diagnosis and management of febrile neutropenia in pediatric oncology patients—a systematic review. Diagnostics (Basel). 2022;12(8):1800.
3. Castagnola E, et al. A prospective study on the epidemiology of febrile episodes during chemotherapy-induced neutropenia in children with cancer or after hematopoietic stem cell transplantation. Clin Infect Dis. 2007 Nov 15;45(10):1296–304.
4. Hao R, Saleh M, Liang T, et al. The prevalence of serious bacterial infections in neutropenic immunocompetent febrile children. Am J Emerg Med. 2021;45:1–6.
5. Nagalapuram V, McCall D, Palabindela P, et al. Outcomes of isolated neutropenia referred to pediatric hematology- oncology clinic. Pediatrics. 2020;146(4):e20193637.
6. Walkovich K, Boxer LA. How to approach neutropenia in childhood. Pediatr Rev. 2013;34:4.
7. Segel GB, Halterman JS. Neutropenia in pediatric practice. Pediatr Rev. 2008;29:12.
8. Grandjean-Blanchet C, et al. Value based care for healthy children with first episode of febrile neutropenia. Hosp Pediatr. 2023;13(6):536–43.

A Patient with a History of Traumatic Brain Injury and Fever

Lucia An, Christopher J. Ferber, and Hanna Siddiqui

1 Case

A 12-year-old female with a history of traumatic brain injury (TBI) 5 years ago with resulting spastic cerebral palsy, cerebrally mediated autonomic dysfunction, ventriculoperitoneal (VP) shunt for hydrocephalus, gastrostomy tube (G-tube) dependence, ventilator dependence, neurogenic bladder, and hypothalamic-pituitary-adrenal (HPA) axis dysfunction presents to the emergency room with emesis and fever for 4 days. Her parents report that she had been uncomfortable for the past 2 days; however, she now appears lethargic. She stays home with her parents, and there has been no recent travel or ill contacts. There have been no changes to her home medications, which include the following: budesonide nebulizer, omeprazole, gabapentin, baclofen, hydrocortisone, and cephalexin for urinary tract infection prophylaxis. She has not tolerated her feeds or medications over the last few days. On review of systems, there is no cough, runny nose, diarrhea, constipation, rash, or other symptoms.

Her initial vitals show a heart rate of 128 bpm, blood pressure of 112/84 mmHg, respiratory rate of 21 breaths/min, and temperature of 99.8 °F. On physical exam, she appears tired with dry mucous membranes. She has no focal neurological deficits, and her VP shunt is palpated along her left parietal region without any tenderness or discontinuity. Her G-tube site is clean without any erythema. The remainder of her exam is within normal limits.

L. An (✉) · H. Siddiqui
Division of Pediatric Hospital Medicine, UCLA Mattel Children's Hospital, Los Angeles, CA, USA
e-mail: lan@mednet.ucla.edu; hannasiddiqui@mednet.ucla.edu

C. J. Ferber
UCLA Mattel Children's Hospital, Los Angeles, CA, USA
e-mail: CJFerber@mednet.ucla.edu

A. Kamzan et al. (eds.), *Children with Medical Complexity in the Emergency Department*, https://doi.org/10.1007/978-3-031-62517-6_4

A complete blood count, comprehensive metabolic panel, urinalysis, upper respiratory viral panel, and blood cultures (aerobic and anaerobic) are collected. A shunt X-ray series is read as normal. A chest X-ray shows no new focal opacities. Empiric intravenous (IV) ceftriaxone and vancomycin are started for presumed sepsis, and the decision to admit the patient is made.

While awaiting admission, the nurse informs the physician that the patient vomited, and vital signs now show a heart rate of 133 bpm, blood pressure of 83/58 mmHg, respiratory rate of 18 breaths/min, and temperature of 101.3 °F. On re-examination, she remains lethargic, has delayed capillary refill time, and tachycardia. Her serum labs are significant for hyponatremia, hypoglycemia, elevated blood urea nitrogen/creatinine ratio, normal complete blood count, and normal liver function tests. Intravenous antibiotics are broadened to cefepime from ceftriaxone, and two normal saline boluses are provided. Nevertheless, after 1 h, she remains tachycardic with borderline low blood pressures unresponsive to normal saline fluids.

2 Discussion Questions

1. What is the next best step in management?
2. What are the complications of the underlying condition?

3 Case Answers

1. This patient has underlying adrenocorticotrophic hormone (ACTH) deficiency from her traumatic brain injury and is presenting in an adrenal crisis. The next step in management would be to provide intravenous steroids at stress dosing, due to concern for central adrenal insufficiency with increased needs during illness and missed doses of her home medications. Additionally, it is important to continue intravenous fluids, monitor vital signs including blood pressure, and perform serial physical exams to determine the need for vasopressors.
2. An untreated adrenal crisis is a life-threatening condition. Patients will deteriorate with hypotension and worsening electrolyte abnormalities without glucocorticoid treatment.

4 Learning Objectives

1. Understand the pathophysiology of adrenal insufficiency.
2. Recognize signs and symptoms of adrenal crisis.
3. Describe the complications of this condition.
4. Understand initial management of adrenal insufficiency.

5 Discussion

Adrenal insufficiency (AI) is a serious condition defined by decreased production of adrenal gland hormones, which include glucocorticoids, mineralocorticoids, and androgens. The basic physiology involves the following: the hypothalamus secretes corticotropin-releasing hormone (CRH) leading to stimulation of the anterior pituitary gland to secrete ACTH, which then acts on the zona fasciculata of the adrenal gland to stimulate secretion of cortisol (Fig. 1). Causes of AI may be divided into primary adrenal insufficiency (PAI), a problem with hormone synthesis at the level of the adrenal glands, and central (secondary) adrenal insufficiency (CAI), a problem with the HPA axis. Although uncommon, adrenal insufficiency is potentially fatal and has variable and nonspecific clinical signs and symptoms, which may delay diagnosis and management. It is therefore crucial for clinicians to have a good understanding of causes, presentation, and management of this condition.

The most common cause of PAI is congenital adrenal hyperplasia (CAH), an autosomal recessive disorder, with an incidence of 1:14,000 to 1:18,000 births [1]. Greater than 90% of cases of CAH are due to a mutation in *CYP21A* [2], coding for 21-hydroxylase enzyme involved in cortisol biosynthesis. Enzyme deficiency leads to a buildup of 17-hydroxyprogesterone (17-OHP), the adrenal precursor which 21-hydroxylase converts to 11-deoxycortisol (Fig. 2). Then, excess 17-OHP accumulates and is shunted into overproduction of androgens causing female newborn virilization. Based on the severity of 21-hydroxylase enzyme deficiency, CAH is divided into classic and non-classic CAH. Classic CAH is further subdivided into "salt wasting" and "simple virilization" forms based on the severity of aldosterone deficiency. The salt wasting form is more severe with profound aldosterone deficiency leading to adrenal crisis within the first couple of weeks of life. The simple virilization form has retained 1–2% aldosterone activity leading to a less severe neonatal presentation [3, 4]. Non-classic CAH is more common and has some preserved enzyme activity causing less severe and variable presentations, perhaps with no salt wasting at all [4].

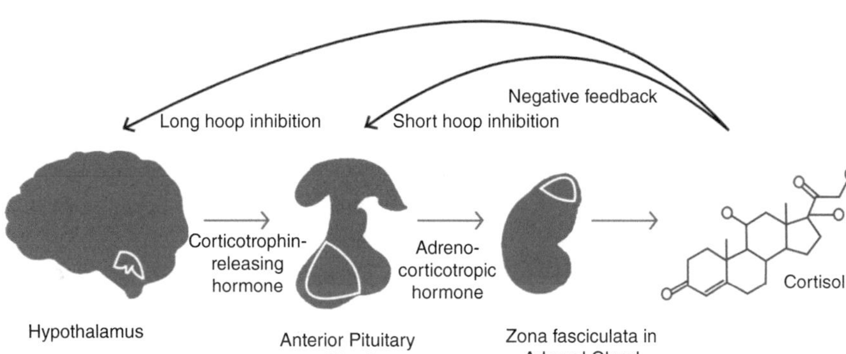

Fig. 1 The hypothalamic-pituitary-adrenal axis

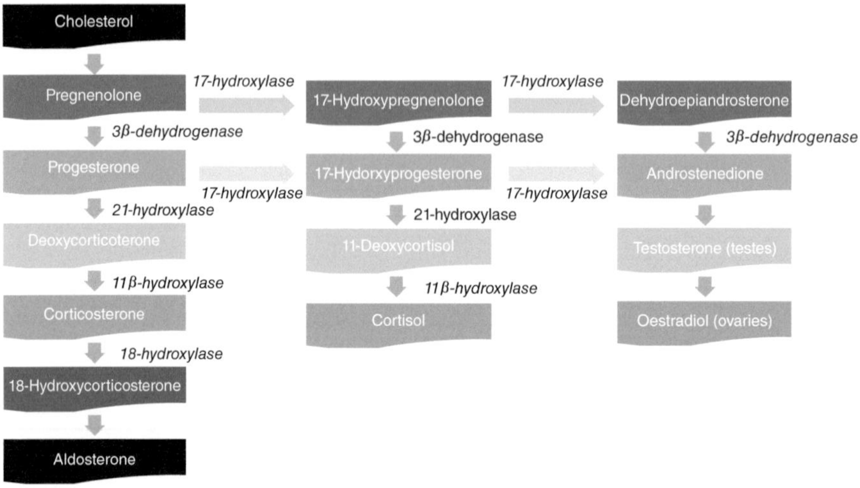

Fig. 2 Adrenal steroidogenesis pathway

The newborn screen measures 17-OHP levels to allow for early diagnosis of CAH caused by 21-OH deficiency. False positives can occur in premature infants, and false negatives can occur if mother has been exposed to glucocorticoids prenatally [3, 5].

In contrast, CAI is due to decreased ACTH production in the anterior pituitary, which subsequently leads to decreased cortisol hormone production. It can be caused by hypothalamic and/or hypopituitary conditions, such as tumors, radiation treatment, surgery, midline defects, and infiltrative diseases. Our case demonstrates CAI due to ACTH deficiency from TBI.

Additionally, chronic steroid use can also lead to CAI through a similar mechanism. Long courses of supraphysiologic exogenous steroids result in suppression of endogenous ACTH production. The lack of stimulation by ACTH further causes ACTH receptors in adrenal tissue to downregulate. If exogenous steroids are then stopped abruptly, the body can no longer mount an adequate ACTH or cortisol response, resulting in CAI. There is limited data in pediatrics regarding the dose threshold and dose duration, which leads to developing steroid-induced adrenal insufficiency [6]. A small study demonstrated that severe adrenal insufficiency seems unlikely at physiological replacement dosing for up to 2 weeks [7]. Notably, those with CAI classically do not have mineralocorticoid deficiency since aldosterone secretion is regulated by the renin-aldosterone system and therefore would not be expected to be at risk of salt wasting. However, hyponatremia can still be seen in CAI through an alternate mechanism. Given that cortisol is a negative feedback hormone to CRH, the CRH levels will increase in cortisol deficiency, which also leads to increased production of antidiuretic hormone (ADH) and absorption of free water, which can cause hyponatremia. Cortisol also directly suppresses the production of ADH [8–10].

An adrenal crisis, which is an acute form of adrenal insufficiency, may be triggered by acute illnesses, surgery, burns, or trauma. The clinical presentation of adrenal crisis due to PAI and CAI shares some similarities due to glucocorticoid deficiency, including hypoglycemia, fatigue, abdominal pain, nausea, and vomiting. PAI will have manifestations of mineralocorticoid deficiency, which includes hypotension, salt craving, hyponatremia, hyperkalemia, and metabolic acidosis.

The differential diagnoses for this patient's presentation include infection, specifically gastroenteritis and urinary tract infection, in a patient with emesis and feeding intolerance. In this medically complex patient, it is important to consider ventilator-associated pneumonia and VP shunt infection. Additionally, when patients are unresponsive to fluids and infection is suspected, consider septic shock. Children in this age group presenting with acute vomiting should also be evaluated for other emergency diagnoses including diabetes ketoacidosis, ovarian or testicular torsion, appendicitis, and hemolytic uremic syndrome. For these differentials, a point-of-care glucose and physical exam will aid diagnosis. Furthermore, abusive head trauma should be considered for a medically complex child presenting with emesis given that this patient population is at risk of maltreatment [11, 12].

Acute management of adrenal crisis involves providing immediate glucocorticoids, normal saline boluses for hypovolemic shock, and monitoring for electrolyte abnormalities including hyperkalemia, hyponatremia, and hypoglycemia. Electrocardiograms are also important if persistent hyperkalemia is seen. Electrolyte derangements will improve with glucocorticoid replacement and intravenous fluids.

For patients with known underlying adrenal insufficiency, empiric stress dose glucocorticoids should be given immediately for the management of adrenal crisis. However, for those with suspected adrenal insufficiency yet no official diagnosis, confirmatory labs, such as an ACTH stimulation test, may be warranted first followed by a stress dose of glucocorticoids. If confirmatory serum labs are unable to be collected and the patient is critically ill, treat empirically and do not delay providing stress dose steroids.

Appropriate hydrocortisone dosing for acute management of adrenal crisis and other potential stressors based on Endocrine Society clinical practice guidelines is described in Table 1 [13].

Table 1 Management of patients on glucocorticoids based on specific conditions

Condition	Medication dosing
Acute adrenal crisis	IV hydrocortisone 50–100 mg/m^2 bolus, followed by repeat dose of hydrocortisone 50–100 mg/m^2/day divided q6h
Major surgery, trauma, or condition requiring intensive care	IV hydrocortisone 50 mg/m^2 followed by hydrocortisone 50–100 mg/m^2 divided q6h
Minor or moderate surgical stress	IM hydrocortisone 50 mg/m^2 or double-triple home hydrocortisone replacement dose

The initial screening step in the laboratory diagnosis of adrenal insufficiency is measurement of serum cortisol in the early morning (between 6 and 8 AM). Early-morning testing is essential because of the diurnal variation in serum cortisol. For patients <6 months of age, the early-morning timing for testing is less important because young infants have not yet developed significant diurnal variation of serum cortisol. A morning serum cortisol of less than 3 μg/dL is concerning, 3–7 μg/dL is equivocal, and greater than 8 μg/dL is reassuring. If basal serum cortisol is low, then an ACTH stimulation test usually should be performed to confirm the diagnosis of adrenal insufficiency. However, ACTH stimulation testing is not always necessary or practical, and the decision to perform this test depends on the clinical scenario. A stimulated serum cortisol of less than 15 μg/dl is diagnostic of AI. The cutoff is based on timing the lab drawn at exactly 60 min. A level drawn too early or late may yield a false-positive result. Both PAI and CAI will have a low cortisol response to an ACTH stimulation test. In PAI, the pathology is at the level of the adrenal gland itself, so ACTH would not be expected to raise cortisol levels. In CAI, baseline lack of ACTH stimulation leads to receptor downregulation, which also results in adrenal glands that are resistant to ACTH stimulation.

Other tests to consider include progesterone, renin, and aldosterone levels as these provide an early and sensitive indicator of mineralocorticoid deficiency. They should be measured in all patients at high risk of acute adrenal crisis. These markers are part of the initial evaluation of newborn infants with suspicion for congenital adrenal hyperplasia (CAH) such as those with atypical genital appearance, positive newborn screen, or hyponatremia and hyperkalemia. These tests may also be helpful for monitoring the adequacy of mineralocorticoid replacement therapy. Measurement of aldosterone and its precursors is most useful for testing for enzymatic defects specific to rare disorders of mineralocorticoid synthesis. As mentioned previously, patients with classic CAH due to 21-hydroxylase have markedly elevated 17-hydroxyprogesterone. Other steroid metabolites are sometimes measured to distinguish between 21-hydroxylase deficiency and other rare forms of CAH. Tests of adrenal androgens (e.g., dehydroepiandrosterone sulfate and androstenedione) and their steroid precursors may be helpful in establishing the diagnosis and type of CAH. Adrenal androgens are elevated in some forms of CAH before treatment is initiated due to disrupted steroid biosynthesis, including classic CAH due to 21-hydroxylase deficiency or 11-beta-hydroxylase deficiency. Adrenal androgens are usually low-normal or subnormal in patients with other forms of adrenal insufficiency, and their measurements are not required for the initial diagnosis [13, 14].

6 Review Questions

1. What is the appropriate stress steroid medication and dosing if there is concern for adrenal crisis?

   (A) 50–100 mg/m^2 dexamethasone
   (B) 50–100 mg/m^2 fludrocortisone

   (C) 50–100 mg/m^2 hydrocortisone
   (D) 50–100 mg/m^2 prednisone

2. What hormone level is elevated in classic CAH?

   (A) 11-Deoxycortisol
   (B) 17-Hydroxypregnenolone
   (C) 17-Hydroxyprogesterone
   (D) Deoxycorticosterone

3. What electrolyte lab abnormalities might you see in adrenal crisis from primary adrenal insufficiency?

   (A) Hypernatremia, hypokalemia
   (B) Hyponatremia, hypokalemia
   (C) Hypernatremia, hyperkalemia
   (D) Hyponatremia, hyperkalemia

7 Answers

1. **C**. 50–100 mg/m^2 hydrocortisone. Hydrocortisone is the preferred agent to treat adrenal crisis and should be administered parenterally. It has the ideal glucocorticoid pharmacokinetics and balance of glucocorticoid and mineralocorticoid effects. Dexamethasone and prednisone require different dosing due to different relative glucocorticoid activity. Fludrocortisone has minimal glucocorticoid activity.
2. **C**. 17-Hydroxyprogesterone. Classic CAH is caused by 21-hydroxylase deficiency, which is an enzyme involved in converting 17-hydroxyprogesterone to 11-deoxycortisol. The precursor, 17-hydroxyprogesterone, is therefore elevated in classic CAH. The hormones 11-deoxycortisol and deoxycorticosterone are elevated in 11-*β* hydroxylase deficiency. The hormone 17-hydroxyprogenolone is elevated in 3*β*-hydroxysteroid dehydrogenase deficiency.
3. **D**. Hyponatremia, hyperkalemia. Primary adrenal insufficiency causes mineralocorticoid deficiency leading to hyponatremia and hyperkalemia. Additionally, hyponatremia is accentuated by cortisol deficiency, which leads to increased ADH secretion.

8 Takeaway Points

1. Adrenal crisis should be on the differential for patients at risk or with a history of PAI or CAI, especially in the setting of stressors such as infection.
2. Untreated adrenal crisis can be fatal. Patients will deteriorate with hypotension and worsening electrolyte abnormalities without glucocorticoid treatment.

3. Clinical presentation of adrenal crisis from PAI and CAI includes hypoglycemia, fatigue, abdominal pain, nausea, and vomiting.
4. PAI will have manifestations of mineralocorticoid deficiency, which includes hypotension, salt craving, hyponatremia, hyperkalemia, and metabolic acidosis.
5. For evaluation, first perform an early-morning serum cortisol. If low, conduct an ACTH stimulation test. Helpful lab tests include progesterone, renin, and aldosterone levels as these provide an early and sensitive indicator of mineralocorticoid deficiency. They are part of initial CAH and acute adrenal crisis evaluations.

References

1. Speiser PW, Arlt W, Auchus RJ, et al. Congenital adrenal hyperplasia due to steroid 21-hydroxylase deficiency: an endocrine society clinical practice guideline. J Clin Endocrinol Metab. 2018;103(11):4043–88. https://doi.org/10.1210/jc.2018-01865.
2. White PC, Speiser PW. Congenital adrenal hyperplasia due to 21-hydroxylase deficiency*. Endocr Rev. 2000;21(3):245–91. https://doi.org/10.1210/edrv.21.3.0398.
3. Turcu AF, Auchus RJ. Adrenal steroidogenesis and congenital adrenal hyperplasia. Endocrinol Metab Clin N Am. 2015;44(2):275–96. https://doi.org/10.1016/j.ecl.2015.02.002.
4. El-Maouche D, Arlt W, Merke DP. Congenital adrenal hyperplasia. Lancet. 2017;390(10108):2194–210. https://doi.org/10.1016/S0140-6736(17)31431-9.
5. Coulm B, Coste J, Tardy V, et al. Efficiency of neonatal screening for congenital adrenal hyperplasia due to 21-hydroxylase deficiency in children born in mainland France between 1996 and 2003. Arch Pediatr Adolesc Med. 2012;166(2):113–20. https://doi.org/10.1001/archpediatrics.2011.774.
6. Akahoshi S, Hasegawa Y. Steroid-induced iatrogenic adrenal insufficiency in children: a literature review. Endocrine. 2020;1(2):125–37. https://doi.org/10.3390/endocrines1020012.
7. Spiegel RJ, Oliff AI, Bruton J, Vigersky RA, Echelberger CK, Poplack DG. Adrenal suppression after short-term corticosteroid therapy. Lancet. 1979;313(8117):630–3. https://doi.org/10.1016/S0140-6736(79)91077-8.
8. Raff H. Glucocorticoid inhibition of neurohypophysial vasopressin secretion. Am J Phys. 1987;252(4 Pt 2):R635–44. https://doi.org/10.1152/ajpregu.1987.252.4.R635.
9. Erkut ZA, Pool C, Swaab DF. Glucocorticoids suppress corticotropin-releasing hormone and vasopressin expression in human hypothalamic neurons. J Clin Endocrinol Metab. 1998;83(6):2066–73. https://doi.org/10.1210/jcem.83.6.4881.
10. Jessani N, Jehangir W, Behman D, Yousif A, Spiler IJ. Secondary adrenal insufficiency: an overlooked cause of hyponatremia. J Clin Med Res. 2015;7(4):286–8. https://doi.org/10.14740/jocmr2041w.
11. Radovick S, Misra M. Pediatric endocrinology: a practical clinical guide. Cham: Springer; 2018.
12. Auron M, Raissouni N. Adrenal insufficiency. Pediatr Rev. 2015;36(3):92–103. https://doi.org/10.1542/pir.36-3-92.
13. Bornstein SR, Allolio B, Arlt W, et al. Diagnosis and treatment of primary adrenal insufficiency: an endocrine society clinical practice guideline. J Clin Endocrinol Metab. 2016;101(2):364–89. https://doi.org/10.1210/jc.2015-1710.
14. Bancos I, Hahner S, Tomlinson J, Arlt W. Diagnosis and management of adrenal insufficiency. Lancet Diabet Endocrinol. 2015;3(3):216–26. https://doi.org/10.1016/s2213-8587(14)70142-1.

Further Reading

Akahoshi S, Hasegawa Y. Steroid-induced iatrogenic adrenal insufficiency in children: a literature review. Endocrines. 2020;1(2):125–37. (Spiegel et al. 1979)

Bethin K, Majumdar I, Mugli L. Chapter 13 Adrenal insufficiency. In: Pediatric endocrinology: a practical clinical guide. Berlin: Springer International Publishing; 2018.

Krone N, Dhir V, Ivison HE, Arlt W. Congenital adrenal hyperplasia and P450 oxidoreductase deficiency. Clin Endocrinol. 2007;66(2):162–72. https://doi.org/10.1111/j.1365-2265.2006.02740.x.

Cloudy Dialysate Effluent and Abdominal Pain in a Patient on Peritoneal Dialysis

Madison Shirkey Anderson and Rose Ayoob

1 Case

A 17-year-old female with end-stage renal disease (ESRD) secondary to focal segmental glomerulosclerosis (FSGS) on peritoneal dialysis (PD) presents to the emergency room. Her family reports cloudy effluent with her initial drain tonight and a fever. For the last 2 days, she has had worsening abdominal pain and nausea. Per the home dialysis unit protocol, the patient collected PD fluid at home after a 2-h dwell and brought the fluid to emergency room. She initially required PD starting at 15 years of age and has minimal residual renal function. She was treated for an exit site infection 1 month prior to presentation. She also has a history of hypertension and metabolic bone disease.

The physical exam includes vital signs as follows: temperature 39.5C, heart rate 135, blood pressure 100/70, and oxygen saturation 99% on room air. The patient's current weight is 50 kg with a dry weight of 45 kg. She is awake and alert but appears uncomfortable. Facial and periorbital edema is noted. She has crackles in both lung bases, but non-labored respiration. She has a "dry abdomen" (meaning no peritoneal effluent is present in the abdomen), diffuse tenderness to palpation, and diminished bowel sounds throughout; the PD catheter exit site is noted to have minimal crusting and erythema.

M. S. Anderson (✉)
Hoops Family Children's Hospital, JCESOM Marshall University, Huntington, WV, USA
e-mail: Andersonmad@marshall.edu

R. Ayoob
Pediatric Nephrology, Hoops Family Children's Hospital, JCESOM Marshall University, Huntington, WV, USA
e-mail: Ayoob1@marshall.edu

A. Kamzan et al. (eds.), *Children with Medical Complexity in the Emergency Department*, https://doi.org/10.1007/978-3-031-62517-6_5

2 Discussion Questions

1. What is the differential diagnosis for cloudy peritoneal effluent?
2. What is the best next step in management after initial ED assessment?
3. What management decisions need to be specially considered in this patient?

3 Case Answers

1. The differential diagnosis of cloudy effluent includes culture-positive infectious peritonitis or infectious peritonitis with sterile cultures; chemical peritonitis; calcium channel blockers; eosinophilia of the effluent; hemoperitoneum (e.g., from menses, trauma); or a specimen taken from a "dry" abdomen. Rarer causes include malignancy and chylous effluent.
2. A detailed history should be obtained, including possible break in sterile technique during home PD, any recent invasive procedures, and change in bowel habits. A physical exam focusing on the abdomen and dialysis catheter site should then follow; the peritoneal fluid should be sent for analysis (including cell count, differential, Gram stain, and culture), and broad-spectrum antibiotics should be administered.
3. PD patients presenting with cloudy effluent should be presumed to have peritonitis and treated as such until proven otherwise. The patient's risk factors for peritonitis, home dialysis management plan, medication dosing adjustment needs and fluid resuscitation needs should be assessed on an individual level.

4 Learning Objectives

1. Understand the clinical evaluation and diagnostic criteria for peritonitis in PD patients.
2. Identify patient, technique, and environment-related risk factors for PD-related peritonitis.
3. Understand management and antibiotic administration in PD-related peritonitis.
4. Evaluate the need for inpatient treatment versus outpatient treatment of PD-related peritonitis.

5 Discussion

There are two primary forms of dialysis utilized in ESRD: hemodialysis (HD) and peritoneal dialysis (PD). In HD, the blood is removed from the body and filtered by a machine before being circulated back to the body. This form of dialysis most often takes place in a hospital 3–5 times per week and requires constant intravenous connection during the procedure, making performing other activities during that time very difficult. Peritoneal dialysis is frequently completed at home on a daily basis. Dialysate fluid is placed into the abdomen through a peritoneal catheter that has previously been surgically placed. The fluid then cleanses the blood through the abdominal wall and is drained after a set dwell time. The removed fluid is referred to as peritoneal effluent or PD fluid.

Peritoneal dialysis (PD) remains the most common form of dialysis initially prescribed to children with ESRD worldwide [1, 2]. As peritoneal dialysis can most often be performed at home by families, it is thought to improve the patient's quality of life as it allows them to make fewer changes to their routines. This encourages ongoing school attendance and family/after-school activities [2]. Although PD serves as an effective means of accomplishing solute and fluid removal, infectious complications frequently occur and often compromise the continued function of the procedure. Peritonitis and catheter exit-site infections are the most common infections, with the rates of these infections routinely demonstrated to be greater in children than in adults [1].

The cause of peritonitis in most cases is not obvious. In a study by the International Pediatric Peritonitis Registry of the 491 episodes of non-fungal peritonitis, 72% had no identifiable cause. In the remainder, the most common causes were touch contamination (12%), exit-site and tunnel infections (7%), and catheter perforation/leakage (2.1%) [1]. The identification of additional risk factors that can increase rates of peritonitis is important to optimize patient outcome. Risk factors may be modifiable or non-modifiable and can be looked at as patient-related, catheter- and exit site-related, and technique-related. Studies have shown that the rate of peritonitis in children is inversely related to age [3]. This may be due to the proximity of the PD exit site to the diaper or to a gastrostomy, vesicostomy, or nephrostomy site. Catheter design and exit-site location are also important factors. The preferred catheter in children, from a peritonitis risk standpoint, is a double-cuff swan-neck catheter with a downward directed exit site as these have been associated with lower infection rates [4]. Prophylactic antibiotics are recommended at the time of PD catheter insertion as well as with reported episodes of intraluminal contamination. Certain invasive procedures such as dental surgery, colonoscopy, or urinary tract-related surgeries are also treated with prophylaxis.

Catheter, exit-site, and tunnel infections are most often due to *Staphylococcus* or *Pseudomonas* and are associated with significant increased risk of peritonitis. Catheter-related infections include both exit-site and tunnel infections. "Exit site" refers to the site where the catheter exits the abdomen, and infections are usually associated with purulent drainage surrounding the area. "Tunnel infection" refers to the subcutaneous portion of the peritoneal catheter and can have symptoms that include overlying erythema, edema, or tenderness over the tunneled catheter [5]. Delaying the start of dialysis to allow wound healing from the PD catheter, as well as proper exit-site care, reduces the risk of infection. In both children and adults on PD, 50–60% of cases of peritonitis are due to Gram-positive organisms and 20–30% are due to Gram-negative organisms. Fungal peritonitis comprises less than 5% of cases [6]. Bacteria can invade the peritoneal cavity through several routes: intraluminal (touch contamination), periluminal (catheter related), transluminal through bowel wall, systemic (hematogenous), and, rarely, ascending through the vagina [6]. Patients, parents, and caregivers need one-on-one training by PD nurse trainers. The goals of training include the ability to safely perform all required PD procedures, ability to both recognize and prevent contamination and infection, and knowledge of the appropriate responses to these complications.

The presentation of peritonitis is often associated with cloudy effluent, but the clinical presentation may vary from asymptomatic to severe illness. Other signs and symptoms include fever, abdominal pain sometimes associated with rebound tenderness, nausea, vomiting, diarrhea, and in severe cases sepsis. Cloudy effluent is present in 98–100% of patients, and therefore this presentation should be treated as peritonitis until proven otherwise [5]. A thorough clinical assessment should include inquiring about a history of possible touch contamination/break in sterile technique during home PD, any recent invasive procedures (dental work, colonoscopy, etc.), or changes in bowel habits (diarrhea or constipation). A physical exam should be performed, focusing on the abdomen and inspection of the dialysis catheter site.

The diagnostic criteria for peritonitis state that it should be considered when at least two of the following are present: (1) clinical features consistent with peritonitis, i.e., abdominal pain and/or cloudy dialysis effluent; (2) dialysis effluent white cell count >100/μL or >0.1 × 10^9/L (after a dwell time of at least 2 h), with >50% polymorphonuclear cells; and (3) positive dialysis effluent culture [7, 8]. If considered, patients should be promptly evaluated and treated.

To prevent delays in treatment, empiric antibiotic therapy is given to cover both Gram-positive and Gram-negative organisms once dialysis effluent is collected and sent for Gram stain, cell count, and culture. Antibiotics are recommended to be administered intraperitoneally to ensure immediate bioavailability; however, if the presentation is consistent with sepsis or systemic illness, intravenous antibiotics should be promptly administered as well. Recommendations for intraperitoneal dosing are available for continuous and intermittent dosing based on the PD prescription. Intravenous antibiotics should take into consideration whether or not the patient has any residual renal function. Typical empiric antibiotic coverage is vancomycin or a first-generation cephalosporin plus a third-generation antibiotic to ensure adequate Gram-positive and Gram-negative coverage. Fourth-generation cephalosporin monotherapy can also be considered [9]. Coverage should be based on a patient's prior cultures, if applicable, and local biogram sensitivities. The patient's dialysis unit should also be contacted for additional guidance and review of unit protocols for the treatment of peritonitis and antibiotic sensitivity patterns. Fluid resuscitation may be necessary but should take into account the patient's current weight relative to their dry weight and whether or not they have any residual renal function, so as to avoid fluid overload.

If cultures result to reveal a bacterial etiology for the infection, antibiotics can then be appropriately narrowed. If the initial culture remains negative at 72 h but the patient's symptoms have improved on empiric therapy, continued broad-spectrum single-therapy coverage can be considered for ongoing 2 weeks of treatment. If the patient fails to improve on empiric therapy, repeat cultures should be considered, and consideration of atypical organisms or fungal infections may need to be considered. After 5 days of failed improvement, catheter removal should be considered. Catheter removal will require dialysis to be temporarily performed via HD, and this decision should be made in conjunction with the patient's nephrology team. In the case of negative cultures and/or failed improvement on broad-spectrum coverage, consultation with the patient's nephrologist and an infectious disease specialist should be considered [7].

Some patients with PD-related peritonitis can be managed on an outpatient basis. When determining the need for inpatient vs. outpatient treatment of peritonitis, certain factors should be considered, including hemodynamic status of the patient and the severity of signs and symptoms. If a patient has fever, concerns for sepsis, or pain difficult to control on oral home medications, the patient should be admitted to the inpatient unit [9]. Additional factors include the dialysis prescription, type of treatment schedule chosen, availability to provide intraperitoneal antibiotics at home, and potential for the patient to have timely follow-up. The patient's home dialysis regimen may need to be modified in order to accommodate the schedule required to administer intraperitoneal antibiotics at home (Fig. 1).

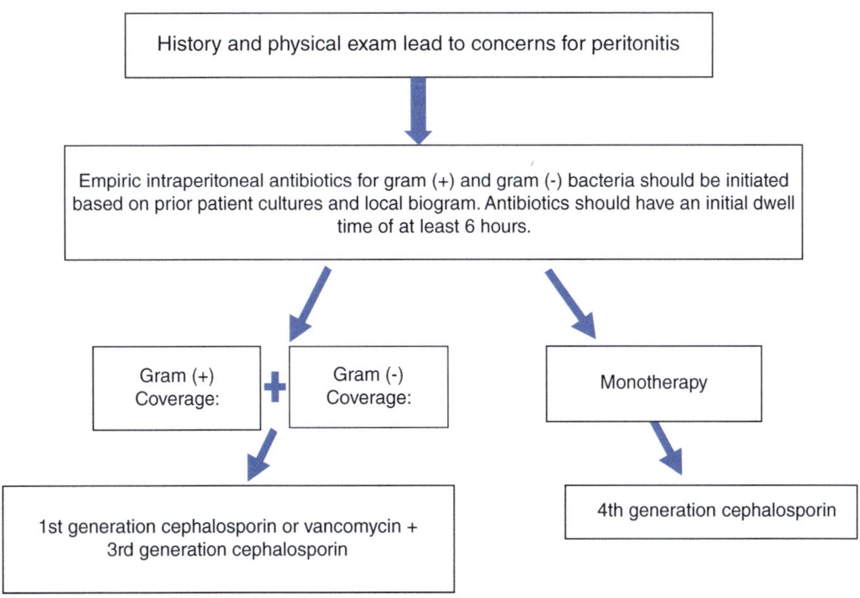

Fig. 1 The algorithm of initial antibiotic management for PD patients presenting with concerns for peritonitis

6 Review Questions

1. The dialysate effluent cell count characteristic of PD-associated bacterial peritonitis is which of the following?
   - (A) Greater than 100/mm^3 WBC with at least 50% PMN
   - (B) Greater than 1000/mm^3 WBC with at least 15% PMN
   - (C) Greater than 50/mm^3 WBC with at least 50% eosinophils
   - (D) Less than 100/mm^3 WBC with more than 50% lymphocytes
2. Catheter exit-site and tunnel infections associated with which of the following organism may predispose to the development of peritonitis?
   - (A) *Klebsiella*
   - (B) *Pseudomonas*
   - (C) *Streptococcus*
   - (D) *Mycoplasma*
3. All of the following are associated with an increased risk for peritonitis, except which of the following?
   - (A) Downward-directed catheter site
   - (B) Single-cuff PD catheter
   - (C) Presence of a gastrostomy tube
   - (D) Exit-site colonization with *Pseudomonas* species
4. Bacteria invade the peritoneal cavity through several routes. Which of the routes listed below is not a common route for PD-associated peritonitis?
   - (A) Transhepatic
   - (B) Hematogenous
   - (C) Enteric
   - (D) Transluminal

7 Answers

1. **A.** Greater than 100/mm^3 WBC with at least 50% PMN. The diagnostic criteria for peritonitis include abdominal pain and/or cloudy dialysis effluent; (2) dialysis effluent white cell count >100/μL or >0.1 × 10^9/L (after a dwell time of at least 2 h), with >50% polymorphonuclear cells; and (3) positive dialysis effluent culture.
2. **B**. *Pseudomonas*. *Staphylococcus* and *Pseudomonas* are associated with an increased risk of peritonitis.
3. **A.** Downward-directed catheter exit site. A downward-directed catheter exit site is associated with a decreased risk of peritonitis. All other answer choices are associated with an increased risk of infection.
4. **A.** Transhepatic. Transhepatic is not a common route for peritonitis. All other options are common routes for infection to spread to the peritoneum.

8 Takeaway Points

1. Peritoneal dialysis-related infections are a significant cause of morbidity and mortality in end-stage chronic kidney disease patients requiring dialysis.
2. Early recognition and treatment are needed to effectively reduce this risk.

References

1. Warady BA, et al. Peritonitis in children who receive long-term peritoneal dialysis: a prospective evaluation of therapeutic guidelines. J Am Soc Nephrol. 2007;18(7):2172–9.
2. Warady BA. Peritoneal dialysis and the pediatric patient. Perit Dial Int. 2012;32(4):393–4.
3. Chadha V, et al. Dialysis-associated peritonitis in children. Pediatr Nephrol. 2010;25(3):425–40.
4. Furth SL, et al. Peritoneal dialysis catheter infections and peritonitis in children: a report of the North American Pediatric Renal Transplant Cooperative Study. Pediatr Nephrol. 2000;15(3–4):179–82.
5. Warady BA, et al. Chapter 14 Peritonitis and exit site infections. In: Pediatric dialysis. 2nd ed. Cham: Springer; 2012. p. 231–56.
6. Szeto CC, Li PK. Peritoneal dialysis-associated peritonitis. Clin J Am Soc Nephrol. 2019;14(7):1100–5.
7. Warady BA, et al. Consensus guidelines for the prevention and treatment of catheter-related infections and peritonitis in pediatric patients receiving peritoneal dialysis: 2012 update. Perit Dial Int. 2012;32(Suppl 2):S32–86.
8. Li PK, et al. ISPD peritonitis recommendations: 2016 update on prevention and treatment. Perit Dial Int. 2016;36(5):481–508.
9. Li PK, et al. ISPD peritonitis guideline recommendations: 2022 update on prevention and treatment. Perit Dial Int. 2022;42(2):110–53.

Respiratory Distress in a Patient with Congenital Heart Disease

Megan M. McKittrick, Laura A. Maitoza, and Mai-King C. Chan

1 Case

A 7-month-old male born at term with prenatally diagnosed hypoplastic left heart syndrome (HLHS) and hypoplastic aortic arch presents to the emergency department (ED). He has undergone palliative surgery with a Norwood/Blalock-Thomas-Taussig (BTT) shunt performed on the day of life 3. He underwent a Glenn procedure with pulmonary arterioplasty and aortic arch reconstruction 10 days ago. He presents today with respiratory distress, worsening cyanosis, and poor feeding. His symptoms developed acutely overnight and have continued to worsen throughout the morning.

Initial vitals in the ED are notable for temperature of 36.9 °C, heart rate of 137 beats per minute (bpm), respiratory rate of 54 breaths per minute, and oxygen saturation of 70% with improvement to 77% on 4 liters per minute (LPM) via nasal cannula. His baseline saturations after his surgeries have been 75–85% on room air. Blood pressure is difficult to obtain, with a most accurate reading of 54/28 mmHg in the left upper extremity. His exam is notable for grunting with subcostal and intercostal retractions. In addition to his baseline perioral cyanosis, he has marked cyanosis of the fingernails bilaterally. A II/VI holosystolic murmur is heard throughout the precordium. Both distal extremities have strong pulses and a capillary refill

M. M. McKittrick (✉)
Department of Pediatrics, UCLA Mattel Children's Hospital, Los Angeles, CA, USA

Division of Pediatric Cardiology, OHSU Doernbecher Children's Hospital, Portland, OR, USA
e-mail: mckittrm@ohsu.edu

L. A. Maitoza · M.-K. C. Chan
Department of Pediatrics, UCLA Mattel Children's Hospital, Los Angeles, CA, USA
e-mail: LMaitoza@mednet.ucla.edu; MCChan@mednet.ucla.edu

A. Kamzan et al. (eds.), *Children with Medical Complexity in the Emergency Department*, https://doi.org/10.1007/978-3-031-62517-6_6

time of 2 seconds. His median sternotomy incision is well healing without erythema or discharge.

He has not missed any doses of his home medications including aspirin 5 mg/kg daily, enalapril 0.2 mg/kg/day divided twice daily, and furosemide 1.5 mg/kg every 8 hours.

1. What is the next best step in management?
2. What workup should be done?
3. What complications should be anticipated?

2 Case Answers

1. Initiate typical supportive care for respiratory distress; escalate to positive-pressure ventilation or intubation if indicated.
2. Initial workup should include a chest radiograph to evaluate for pericardial and/or pleural effusion. Echocardiogram (if available) should be obtained to evaluate cardiac function, outflow tract, Glenn patency, and effusions. A 12-lead electrocardiogram (ECG) may help differentiate between sinus tachycardia secondary to distress and an underlying dysrhythmia. Blood pressure should be repeated on the right upper extremity as prior vascular work can lead to inaccurate readings. Initial labs should include hematocrit, electrolytes, renal function tests, and brain natriuretic peptide (BNP). If effusion or pericarditis is suspected, troponins may be trended.
3. Following Norwood procedure, anticipate cardiac arrest, respiratory arrest, shunt thrombosis, dysrhythmia, and infection [1]. Complications following a bidirectional Glenn include pleural, pericardial, and/or chylous effusions; dysrhythmia; respiratory compromise; and Glenn obstruction [2, 3]. Fontan complications are similar to those post-Glenn and include cyanosis and effusions, as well as longer term complications of hepatic dysfunction, plastic bronchitis, and protein-losing enteropathy [4].

3 Case Continued

After respiratory stabilization, initial chest radiography reveals cardiomegaly with bilateral obscuration of the costophrenic angles (Fig. 1). Limited POCUS shows patent flow through the bidirectional Glenn, with a large circumferential pericardial effusion and diminished systolic function (Fig. 2). An ECG shows sinus tachycardia. He is admitted for urgent pericardiocentesis.

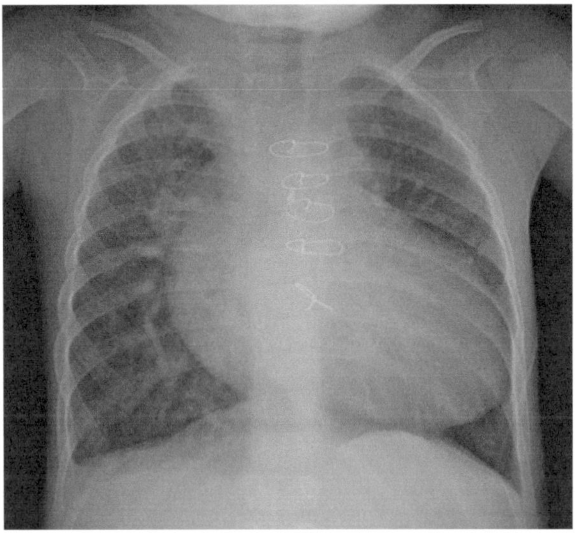

Fig. 1 Chest radiograph demonstrating significant cardiomegaly

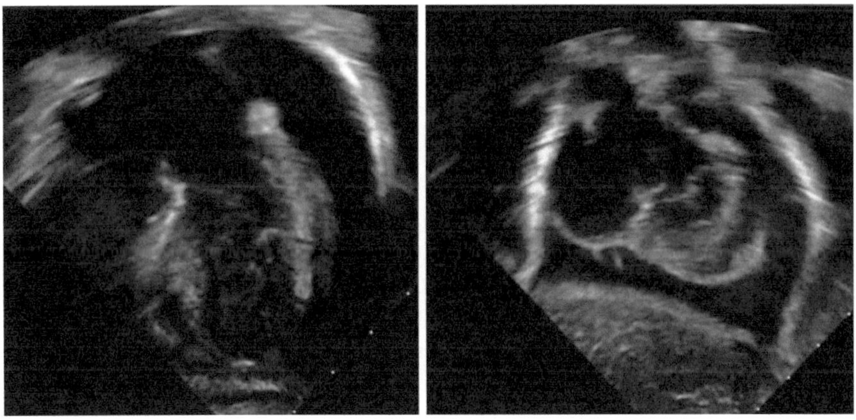

Fig. 2 Bedside POCUS demonstrating pericardial effusion

4 Learning Objectives

1. Understand the pathophysiology of single-ventricle circulation.
2. Describe the expected post-Glenn complications.
3. Understand the initial ED management of pleural effusions in patients with single-ventricle defects.

5 Discussion

5.1 Pathophysiology and Epidemiology

Congenital heart disease (CHD) is one of the most commonly encountered birth defects. Each year, approximately 1.35 million newborns are affected worldwide [5]. Single-ventricle defects are those in which a child is dependent upon a single functional ventricle for both pulmonary and systemic circulation. These lesions include hypoplastic left heart syndrome (HLHS), valvular atresias (i.e., tricuspid or pulmonary atresia), double-outlet right ventricle, double-inlet left ventricle, and unbalanced atrioventricular canal defects. In some instances, two ventricles exist, but flow through the atrioventricular valve(s) enters one predominant ventricle. Single-ventricle defects account for a small subset of congenital lesions; HLHS, the most common single-ventricle defect, comprises 2% of all CHD diagnoses [6].

The majority of single-ventricle lesions are diagnosed via prenatal imaging [7]. In single-ventricle physiology, either systemic or pulmonary circulation is dependent on a patent ductus arteriosus (PDA). As the PDA closes in the neonatal period, the vast majority of single-ventricle lesions are fatal without immediate intervention [8]. The PDA can be maintained using prostaglandin E1 as a temporizing measure while awaiting surgical intervention. The specifics of surgical management for single-ventricle pathology vary on a case-by-case basis, yet the overarching approach is a three-stage palliation process (Fig. 3).

The first stage, the Norwood procedure, is typically performed within the first week of life. A neo-aorta is created by separating the native pulmonary trunk from the left and right portions of the pulmonary artery and joining it with the native ascending aorta. An atrial septectomy is also performed to allow unobstructed pulmonary venous return to the right ventricle. The Norwood is combined with either a Sano or a Blalock-Thomas-Taussig (BTT) shunt. The Sano provides a direct conduit from the right ventricle to the pulmonary artery, while the BTT shunt directs flow from the brachiocephalic trunk (typically the subclavian artery) to the pulmonary artery. The Norwood/Sano or Norwood/BTT aim to create unobstructed systemic blood flow and control the amount of pulmonary circulation.

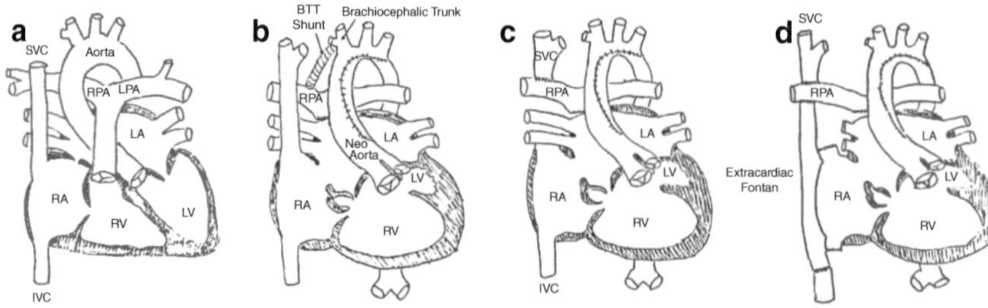

Fig. 3 Normal cardiac anatomy (**a**). The first stage Norwood procedure creates a neo-aorta, atrial septectomy, and BTT shunt with conduit from the brachiocephalic trunk to RPA (**b**). Second stage BCPS involves BTT shunt takedown and anastomosis of the SVC to the RPA (**c**). The third stage Fontan completes the cavopulmonary connection with anastomosis of the IVC to the RPA (**d**)

The second stage, the bidirectional Glenn procedure (also referred to as a bidirectional cavopulmonary shunt, or BCPS), occurs between 4 and 8 months of life. The distal superior vena cava (SVC) is anastomosed to the right pulmonary artery (RPA), while the residual Sano or BTT shunt is taken down. This provides a superior cavopulmonary connection. The primary purpose of the bidirectional Glenn is to reduce the volume load of the single functional ventricle through creation of passive pulmonary circulation.

The third and final palliative stage, the Fontan procedure, provides an inferior cavopulmonary connection from the inferior vena cava (IVC) to the pulmonary artery. This augments the superior connection established by the bidirectional Glenn in the preceding stage. The result is a total cavopulmonary connection with reliance on passive venous return from the systemic vascular beds to the pulmonary vascular beds. This allows for essentially normal oxygenation. Following the Fontan, oxygen saturations are expected to improve to normal values ($SpO_2 > 90\%$).

5.2 *Clinical Presentation and Differential Diagnosis*

The periods between palliative stages remain high risk for patients with single-ventricle physiology, with multiple anticipated complications [8]. It is estimated that up to 80% of affected children present to the emergency department while awaiting their Fontan procedure and tend to have high-acuity chief complaints when compared to their unaffected counterparts [9, 10]. Here, we will focus on complications and diagnostic considerations of pediatric patients presenting for emergency evaluation following bidirectional Glenn palliation.

5.2.1 Effusion

In the case above, the infant presents following a bidirectional Glenn with interval development of a postoperative pericardial effusion. Any infant status post single-ventricle palliation who presents with respiratory compromise, with or without evidence of impaired cardiac output, should raise a high level of suspicion for pericardial or pleural effusion. One of the most commonly encountered complications, effusions affect up to 25% of patients following palliation, most often after bidirectional Glenn. The mechanism is thought to be secondary to increased pressures of the Glenn circuit, driving fluid to collect in the pericardium and pleura. When identified on ultrasound or chest X-ray, initial treatment is drainage via thoracostomy tube placement and/or pericardiocentesis in conjunction with increased diuresis.

5.2.2 Thrombus

Shunts and conduits remain an integral part of single-ventricle physiology and palliation, but pose an inherent risk of thrombosis. Following the Norwood, a thrombus in a Sano or BTT shunt can present as sustained desaturations, respiratory distress, and absence of or decrease in the patient's typical murmur secondary to diminished turbulent flow through the affected shunt. Following the Glenn, thrombi can develop within the SVC to RPA anastomosis. This is secondary to the turbulent venous flow through the anastomosis. Patients should be maintained on anticoagulation such as antiplatelet agents (e.g., aspirin or clopidogrel), vitamin K antagonists (e.g., warfarin), or antithrombotic agents (e.g., enoxaparin). Any concerns for thrombus should prompt urgent ultrasonography to assess Glenn patency as well as a thorough history to elucidate any recent anticoagulation changes. This patient population is at high risk for gut ischemia and necrotizing enterocolitis (NEC). Therefore, it is not uncommon to see anticoagulation modifications in the setting of any recent bloody stool output.

5.2.3 Pulmonary Arterial Hypertension

Pulmonary arterial hypertension (PAH), while not a direct consequence of Glenn circulation, has significant hemodynamic effects if concomitantly present in a palliated patient. Elevated pulmonary arterial pressures and the corresponding increase in pulmonary vascular resistance limit passive forward flow through the Glenn, leading to hypoxia and insufficient development of pulmonary vasculature. PAH presents with sustained desaturations, respiratory distress, hypercapnia, and a mixed metabolic and respiratory acidosis. Lung compliance is often decreased, which can present with marked impairment in chest wall movement. This decrease in compliance may be observed during attempts at bag-mask ventilation. The risk of developing PAH is typically highest in the immediate postoperative period. Treatment is inhaled nitric oxide (iNO) and is oftentimes initiated prophylactically following single-ventricle palliation. Some may be discharged home with pulmonary vasodilators, such as sildenafil or bosentan.

5.2.4 Glenn Obstruction

Any obstruction affecting the Glenn circuit will limit forward pulmonary flow. These include SVC stenosis, PA confluence stenosis, stenosis at the SVC-PA anastomosis, or thrombosis of the Glenn circuit. Patients will present with rapid deterioration including desaturations, respiratory failure, and evidence of SVC syndrome. Initial management in the ED should include volume expansion through intravenous fluid administration. If unstable, heparin can be started for immediate anticoagulation. Definitive treatment is decompression of the obstruction, typically in the cardiac catheterization lab via balloon and/or stent angioplasty.

5.2.5 Systemic Outflow Obstruction

In contrast to Glenn circuit obstruction, systemic outflow obstruction will present with evidence of poor end-organ perfusion, diminished pulses, hypotension, and shock. Common causes include pericardial effusion, re-coarctation of the aorta, and ventricular outflow tract obstruction. Initial ED management should include volume expansion and initiation of vasoactive medications if hemodynamically unstable.

5.2.6 Additional Considerations

Other diagnoses to consider include systolic dysfunction, atrioventricular valve regurgitation, arrhythmia, venovenous and/or aortopulmonary collateral formation, typical postoperative complications (e.g., urinary tract infections, pneumonia), respiratory tract infections (upper and lower), and gastrointestinal infections. Of note, endocarditis should be considered for any febrile patient with CHD and a palliative shunt or conduit who has recently undergone dental work, invasive airway placement, or skin/soft tissue infection with or without appropriate SBE prophylaxis.

5.3 *Management Pearls*

In addition to the complications outlined above, two special considerations exist for emergency management of this patient population:

5.3.1 Blood Pressure

Blood pressure (BP) should be measured on both upper extremities on initial assessment. BP should be assessed according to age-appropriate mean arterial pressure (MAP) goals. If measurements in one extremity are consistently hypotensive without clinical signs of decreased perfusion or hypovolemia, measurements should be repeated on the opposing extremity and/or lower extremities (LEs). Many patients with CHD have aberrant vasculature or have undergone cardiac catheterization or aortic reconstruction, all of which alter vascular hemodynamics. In these cases, collateral vessels are often present, causing the measured BP to be inaccurate and typically lower than true systemic pressures.

BP readings that remain consistently hypotensive in both upper extremities raise concern for tamponade secondary to effusion, which affects contractility and obstructs cardiac output. Such patients should undergo immediate POCUS/echocardiography.

5.3.2 Oxygen Therapy

Oxygen supplementation, when indicated, is typically safe and effective for emergency management of respiratory distress or failure in single-ventricle physiology. In the case of postoperative effusion or atelectasis, oxygen improves desaturations and can be used to achieve a goal saturation range (typically 75–85% post-Norwood and Glenn; >90% post-Fontan). Additionally, oxygen can be used as a pulmonary vasodilator to reduce pulmonary vascular resistance and improve passive Glenn flow.

Oxygen should only be avoided in patients with a documented surgical history of Norwood/BTT shunt or stage I hybrid procedure with PDA stenting and concern for loose pulmonary artery banding. In these cases, pulmonary and systemic circulations are perfused in parallel. Pulmonary over-circulation and systemic hypoperfusion can occur from decreased pulmonary vascular resistance or increased systemic vascular resistance [11]. Oxygen supplementation leads to pulmonary vasodilation, thereby decreasing pulmonary vascular resistance. Resultant pulmonary "steal" can occur, leading to worsening pulmonary over-circulation and signs of systemic hypoperfusion. Any child with a corresponding surgical history should receive oxygen supplementation cautiously or after discussion with a pediatric cardiologist. If the status of the pulmonary bands is unknown, suspect loose bands when patients report a history of worsening tachypnea, cough, and poor feeding. In patients without an obviously contributory surgical risk, pulmonary steal should be suspected when a patient receiving supplemental oxygen develops worsening tachypnea, rales on pulmonary auscultation, edema on chest X-ray, and signs of systemic hypoperfusion (worsening hypotension, oliguria, lactic acidosis).

6 Review Questions

1. A 6-month-old infant with hypoplastic left heart syndrome who had undergone Norwood/Sano in the neonatal period followed by bidirectional Glenn palliation 10 days ago presents with increased work of breathing to ED. She was discharged from the hospital 2 days ago with aspirin and furosemide. Initial vital signs include temperature of 36.5 °C, heart rate of 155 bpm, right upper extremity blood pressure of 80/50 mmHg, and oxygen saturation of 74% on room air. Saturations improve to 82% with 2 L/min nasal cannula. A chest X-ray is obtained.

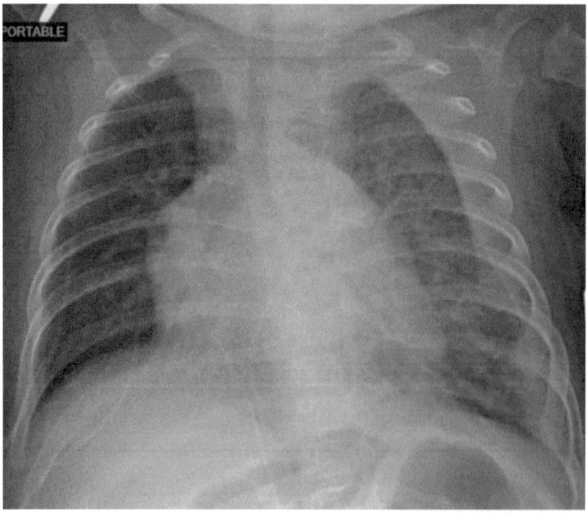

What is the next best step in management?

(A) Obtain intravenous (IV) access, and administer furosemide 1 mg/kg.
(B) Obtain IV access and administer normal saline bolus 20 ml/kg.
(C) Perform thoracostomy with chest tube placement.
(D) Start inhaled nitric oxide via nasal cannula.

2. A 12-month-old infant with tricuspid atresia with normally related great arteries and hypoplastic right ventricle presents to the ED with hypoxia. He is afebrile with oxygen saturation of 68% on room air. He is status post a Glenn procedure with oversewing of the pulmonary valve. His medications include aspirin daily.

What is the next best step in management?

(A) Obtain IV access with labs including complete blood count, comprehensive metabolic panel, coagulation tests, and lactate.
(B) Obtain chest radiograph.
(C) Consult cardiology for formal echocardiogram.
(D) All of the above.

3. A 2-month-old infant with hypoplastic left heart syndrome who has undergone a Norwood with modified Blalock-Taussig-Thomas (BTT) shunt presents with a 1-day history of vomiting, diarrhea, and fever. Two days ago, her brother presented with similar symptoms and was diagnosed with viral gastroenteritis. She appears mottled with capillary refill time of 4 s. Initial vital signs include temperature of 38 °C, heart rate of 185 bpm, right upper extremity blood pressure of 65/30 mmHg, and oxygen saturation of 68% on room air. What is the next best step in management?

(A) Obtain IV access, and administer normal saline bolus 10 mL/kg.
(B) Start oxygen via nasal cannula for hypoxia.
(C) Obtain echocardiogram to rule out shunt obstruction.
(D) Obtain abdominal radiograph to rule out necrotizing enterocolitis (NEC).

4. A 9-year-old child with double-inlet left ventricle that has undergone lateral tunnel Fontan palliation presents to clinic with a 2-day history of decreased exercise tolerance. Her only medication is aspirin daily. Her lab work shows normal complete blood count with hemoglobin of 14 g/dL, normal electrolyte panel, and normal hepatic function panel. Her last cardiology visit was 2 months ago with normal function on echocardiogram. Her vital signs are as follows: temperature 37 °C, heart rate 120 bpm, blood pressure 95/65 mmHg, and oxygen saturation 95% on room air. An electrocardiogram (ECG) is obtained and shown below:

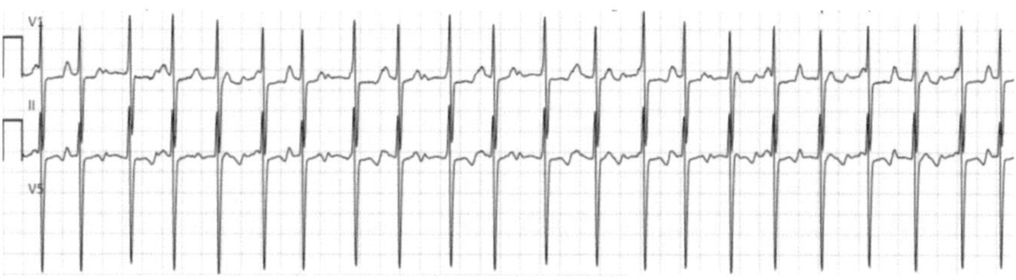

What is the likely diagnosis in this patient?

(A) Acute on chronic heart failure
(B) Protein-losing enteropathy
(C) Atrial flutter
(D) Fontan obstruction

5. A 12-year-old child with double-inlet left ventricle status post lateral tunnel Fontan palliation as a toddler presents to the emergency department with complaint of chest pain. Two days ago, she underwent a cardiac catheterization with coiling of aortopulmonary collaterals and placement of a left pulmonary artery stent for left pulmonary artery stenosis. Her vital signs are unremarkable with normal work of breathing and no murmurs, rubs, or gallops. Her chest pain improves with pain medication. A screening troponin level is normal. An electrocardiogram (ECG) is obtained and is unchanged from a previous clinic ECG.

   What is the likely source of chest pain?

   (A) Non-ST-elevation myocardial infarction
   (B) Referred pain post-catheterization procedure
   (C) Acute pulmonary embolism (PE)
   (D) Acute pericarditis

7 Answers

1. **A**. Obtain intravenous (IV) access, and administer furosemide 1 mg/kg. The above chest X-ray shows a moderate left pleural effusion in a patient that is post-operative from a Glenn procedure. Given that the patient is already on oral furosemide, the next best step is to start an IV diuretic regimen. Inhaled nitric oxide would lower pulmonary artery pressures and encourage more Glenn flow but would not address the primary problem. Chest tube placement would be the next step if diuresis fails. A normal saline bolus could be indicated for signs of dehydration, but would start with 10 ml/kg to avoid worsening effusions.
2. **D**. All of the above. Blood work will help to rule out anemia as a cause for hypoxia or elevated lactate to suggest decreased systemic perfusion. A chest radiograph should be done to evaluate for effusion, pneumothorax, or cardiomegaly. Consult cardiology for formal echocardiogram to rule out a structural abnormality such as significant mitral regurgitation, ventricular dysfunction, or Glenn/SVC obstruction. While awaiting a formal consult, limited POCUS can be performed to evaluate for any significant fluid collection or function abnormality.
3. **A**. Obtain IV access, and administer normal saline bolus 10 mL/kg. This patient likely has viral gastroenteritis. Given her cardiac history, vomiting, tachycardia, desaturations, and slow capillary refill time, the next best step would be administration of a 5–10 mL/kg fluid bolus. Low intravascular volume contributes to

hypoxia by decreasing systemic vascular resistance (SVR) and decreasing shunt flow to pulmonary arteries. Caution should be used when administering oxygen to an infant with a BTT shunt as it can cause pulmonary vasodilation, leading to lower pulmonary vascular resistance (PVR) and pulmonary over-circulation. Shunt obstruction would lead to a more significant degree of desaturation than seen in this case. Infants with shunt physiology are at risk for bowel ischemia in the setting of decreased SVR and decreased gut perfusion; however, NEC typically presents with multiple episodes of bloody stool in the absence of a sick contact.

4. **C**. Atrial flutter. This arrhythmia can be seen following the Fontan procedure as suture lines in the common atria create an abnormal electrical focus. This patient has a high chance of developing heart failure with ventricular dysfunction over the course of her lifetime. However, her recent echocardiogram showed normal function, making heart failure unlikely in this current presentation. Protein-losing enteropathy is often seen in patients following a Fontan. This complication presents with bloating, ascites, and poor weight gain. Routine clinic follow-up should include screening for protein-losing enteropathy. Fontan obstruction is unlikely in this particular case, given a normal oxygen saturation.
5. **B**. Referred pain post-catheterization procedure. The child's pain is likely due to post-procedure pain, which may last up to 5 days after the catheterization. It is best treated with over-the-counter analgesics and supportive care. Acute myocardial infarction is uncommon in this patient population and less likely with a normal troponin. Acute PE can occur after cardiac catheterization, but is unlikely in the absence of new hypoxia or respiratory distress. Of note, should computed tomography angiography be needed to rule out PE, a patient that has undergone a Fontan procedure would need both upper and lower extremity IV access to deliver contrast via both SVC and IVC connections to the pulmonary arteries. Acute pericarditis is unlikely as her vitals, cardiac exam, and ECG are unchanged from her baseline.

8 Takeaway Points

1. Children with single-ventricle defects typically undergo a three-staged palliative surgery course. The periods between surgeries are high risk for morbidity and mortality, with the majority of patients seeking care in the ED at least once in this period.
2. Surgical palliation separates pulmonary and systemic circulations into two parallel circulations, whereby pulmonary circulation is reliant on passive flow.
3. The most common postoperative complications immediately following BCPS include pleural and pericardial effusions, hypoxemia with inadequate pulmonary blood flow, and cardiac arrest.

References

1. Hornik CP, He X, Jacobs JP, et al. Complications after the Norwood operation: an analysis of The Society of Thoracic Surgeons Congenital Heart Surgery Database. Ann Thorac Surg. 2011;92(5):1734–40. https://doi.org/10.1016/j.athoracsur.2011.05.100.
2. Menon SC, McCandless RT, Mack GK, et al. Clinical outcomes and resource use for infants with hypoplastic left heart syndrome during bidirectional Glenn: summary from the Joint Council for Congenital Heart Disease National Pediatric Cardiology Quality Improvement Collaborative registry. Pediatr Cardiol. 2013;34(1):143–8. https://doi.org/10.1007/s00246-012-0403-8.
3. Choi RS, DiNardo JA, Brown ML. Superior cavopulmonary connection: its physiology, limitations, and anesthetic implications. Semin Cardiothorac Vasc Anesth. 2020;24(4):337–48. https://doi.org/10.1177/1089253220939361.
4. Martino D, Rizzardi C, Vigezzi S, et al. Long-term management of Fontan patients: The importance of a multidisciplinary approach. Front Pediatr. 2022;10:886208. https://doi.org/10.3389/fped.2022.886208. Published 2022 Aug 25.
5. GBD 2017 Congenital Heart Disease Collaborators. Global, regional, and national burden of congenital heart disease, 1990–2017: a systematic analysis for the Global Burden of Disease Study 2017 [published correction appears in Lancet Child Adolesc Health. 2020 Feb 7]. Lancet Child Adolesc Health. 2020;4(3):185–200. https://doi.org/10.1016/S2352-4642(19)30402-X.
6. Liu Y, Chen S, Zühlke L, et al. Global birth prevalence of congenital heart defects 1970–2017: updated systematic review and meta-analysis of 260 studies. Int J Epidemiol. 2019;48(2):455–63. https://doi.org/10.1093/ije/dyz009.
7. Roeleveld PP, Axelrod DM, Klugman D, Jones MB, Chanani NK, Rossano JW, Costello JM. Hypoplastic left heart syndrome: from fetus to fontan. Cardiol Young. 2018;28:1275–88. https://doi.org/10.1017/S104795111800135X.
8. Rao PS. Management of congenital heart disease: state of the art-part II-cyanotic heart defects. Children (Basel). 2019;6(4):54. https://doi.org/10.3390/children6040054. Published 2019 Apr 4.
9. Prentice E, Morey N, Richards K, Mastropietro CW. Emergency department use after stage II palliation for children with single ventricle lesions. Pediatr Emerg Care. 2015;31(5):343–7. https://doi.org/10.1097/PEC.0000000000000423.
10. Cashen K, Gupta P, Lieh-Lai M, Mastropietro C. Infants with single ventricle physiology in the emergency department: are physicians prepared? J Pediatr. 2011;159(2):273–7. https://doi.org/10.1016/j.jpeds.2011.01.031.
11. Rychik J, Bush DM, Spray TL, Gaynor JW, Wernovsky G. Assessment of pulmonary/systemic blood flow ratio after first-stage palliation for hypoplastic left heart syndrome: development of a new index with the use of Doppler echocardiography. J Thorac Cardiovasc Surg. 2000;120(1):81–7. https://doi.org/10.1067/mtc.2000.106840.

Further Reading

Rao PS. Management of congenital heart disease: state of the art-part II-cyanotic heart defects. Children (Basel). 2019;6(4):54. https://doi.org/10.3390/children6040054. Published 2019 Apr 4.

Roeleveld PP, Axelrod DM, Klugman D, Jones MB, Chanani NK, Rossano JW, Costello JM. Hypoplastic left heart syndrome: from fetus to fontan. Cardiol Young. 2018;28:1275–88. https://doi.org/10.1017/S104795111800135X.

Salik I, Mehta B, Ambati S. Bidirectional Glenn Procedure or Hemi-Fontan. In: StatPearls. Treasure Island, FL: StatPearls Publishing; 2022.

An Infant with Prolonged Fever, Splenomegaly, and Rash

Evan Wiley

1 Case

A 10-month-old previously healthy fully vaccinated female presents to the emergency department with 8 days of fever. Her parents report that she has been irritable and fatigued with decreased appetite. She is otherwise interacting normally with her parents. She has had no sick contacts and is not in daycare. The family has not travelled or had any animal exposures. Her temperature is 103.7 °F, heart rate is 175 bpm, and blood pressure is 76/48 mmHg. On physical exam, she is ill appearing and pale, and you note the spleen edge 4 cm below the costal margin. She appears irritable, but her mental status is otherwise normal. She has multiple small, mobile cervical lymph nodes and a faint maculopapular rash on her abdomen and back. She has no conjunctivitis, changes to the hands or feet, or changes to the lips or mouth. She has full range of motion of all joints and no joint swelling or pain. Her heart rate is elevated, but heart sounds are normal. Initial labs are notable for a white blood cell count of 9.1×10^9/L, platelet count of 53×10^9/L, hemoglobin of 6.7 g/dL, aspartate transaminase of 372 IU/L, alanine transaminase of 419 IU/L, total bilirubin of 1.6 mg/dL, C-reactive protein of 68 mg/L, and erythrocyte sedimentation rate of 1 mm/hr. Blood and urine cultures are sent. You suspect hemophagocytic lymphohistiocytosis (HLH) and add on a ferritin level, which is 6529 ng/mL.

E. Wiley (✉)
Department of Pediatrics, Cedars-Sinai Medical Center, Los Angeles, CA, USA
e-mail: evan.wiley@cshs.org

A. Kamzan et al. (eds.), *Children with Medical Complexity in the Emergency Department*, https://doi.org/10.1007/978-3-031-62517-6_7

2 Discussion Questions

1. What are the next best steps in management?
2. What complications is she at risk for?
3. What should be the patient's disposition?

3 Case Answers

1. Initial steps should focus on stabilization, furthering the diagnostic evaluation and patient disposition. Initial stabilization should include secure vascular access, fluid resuscitation, and broad-spectrum antibiotics. Measurement of coagulation factors and chest X-ray to evaluate for a mediastinal mass is indicated. Lumbar puncture and brain MRI should be considered following stabilization.
2. Possible complications of HLH include shock, anemia, bleeding from coagulopathy and thrombocytopenia, encephalopathy, respiratory failure, renal failure, and posterior reversible encephalopathy syndrome.
3. The patient will require the care of pediatric specialists in infectious diseases, oncology, and rheumatology. Given the high risk of rapid decompensation, she should be cared for at an institution with a pediatric intensive care unit. For many hospitals, this will require transfer to another institution.

4 Learning Objectives

1. Know how to recognize HLH and send initial testing.
2. Recognize the possible complications of HLH and their evaluation and treatment.
3. Understand the broad range of conditions which may cause or mimic HLH.

5 Discussion

The patient in this case most likely has HLH, a rapidly progressive, highly dangerous disorder of immune hyperactivation in which white blood cells, particularly macrophages, natural killer cells, and cytotoxic T cells, attack the body's own tissues. This immune hyperactivation induces a cytokine storm and systemic inflammation. All of this results in damage to and dysfunction of multiple organ systems.

HLH occurs in roughly 1 in 100,000 pediatric patients without sex predilection. It can present at any age but is most common in children less than 18 months and especially those younger than 3 months. Older patients with HLH are more likely to have an underlying condition triggering HLH, while younger patients are more likely to have a genetic predisposition. Some cases of HLH are familial. Patients with HLH may have a single disease course or relapsing episodes. Without treatment, average life expectancy is less than 1 month after disease onset, and the 1-year survival rate is 5%. With the current treatment regimen, the 6-year survival rate is approximately 50%, though rates vary according to etiology. Patients who have an oncologic cause typically have worse outcomes. The biggest barrier to timely treatment is a delay in diagnosis, which occurs when HLH is not considered on the differential due to its relative rarity; it is not uncommon for HLH to be diagnosed postmortem.

A wide range of underlying conditions may trigger HLH in patients with or without a genetic predisposition. The most common trigger for HLH is viral infection. Many different viruses have been implicated, including Epstein-Barr virus, cytomegalovirus, human immunodeficiency virus, herpes simplex virus, measles, varicella-zoster, and others. Bacterial and fungal infections are less commonly triggers but should be considered, especially in immunosuppressed patients. Malignancies can cause HLH, though it is more common in lymphoid malignancies than solid tumors. Many patients with oncologic causes of HLH have a concurrent viral trigger, so the detection of a viral infection does not preclude the presence of a malignancy. Congenital or acquired immunodeficiencies and immunosuppression are also causes of HLH. When HLH is caused by a rheumatologic disorder, it is referred to as macrophage activation syndrome (MAS). While many rheumatologic disorders may cause MAS, juvenile idiopathic arthritis (JIA) is most strongly associated.

HLH is a syndromic condition, and there is no single universal sign, symptom, or lab result which confirms the presence of HLH [1]. Persistent fever is a key hallmark in the vast majority of cases, though recurrent fever of unknown origin may also occur. Hepatomegaly, splenomegaly, or both are also key signs of HLH. Other history may be nonspecific or reflect organ dysfunction. For example, patients with hepatitis may present with jaundice, while those with encephalopathy may have altered mentation. Other symptoms may include bleeding, rash, seizures, ataxia, and diarrhea. Patients may present in shock and are frequently tachycardic from fever, pain, anemia, dehydration, vasodilatation, or a combination of factors. Patients will often appear ill. Lymphadenopathy or edema may also be present. Rarely, patients may present with renal or respiratory dysfunction, which in severe cases may require dialysis or intubation, respectively. In the absence of end-organ damage, physical exam findings may be nonspecific.

In an ill-appearing patient with high fever, it is often the initial lab results that spark suspicion of HLH. In particular, the presence of a bicytopenia in which two cell lines are diminished (most often anemia and thrombocytopenia though leukopenia or neutropenia may occur) should raise the specter of HLH. Elevated liver enzymes and hyperbilirubinemia are also common findings, reflecting hepatitis, as is coagulopathy and hypofibrinogenemia. C-reactive protein is often elevated, while erythrocyte sedimentation rate may be paradoxically low, especially in MAS, due to hypofibrinogenemia. When HLH is being considered, a ferritin level should be sent immediately. HLH causes markedly elevated ferritin levels, nearly always over 500 ng/mL and often in the thousands, with higher levels being more specific for HLH. Particularly in children, there are few other inflammatory conditions which cause such high levels of ferritin, though systemic JIA may do so with or without MAS. Interpretation of ferritin is difficult in patients who have received many transfusions, which include some patients with cancers at risk for HLH. Markedly high levels of CD25 (soluble interleukin-2 receptor alpha) is highly specific for HLH, but a result may not be available quickly. Lactate dehydrogenase and triglycerides are often elevated as well. Formal diagnostic criteria have undergone minor revisions several times, but commonly used criteria are shown in Table 1. Diagnostic studies should be completed as urgently as possible when HLH is suspected.

In cases where suspicion for HLH is high, serial testing may be needed for patients to meet diagnostic criteria. Also, some of the required tests are likely to have a long turnaround time, and patients with HLH can deteriorate rapidly. Accordingly, a presumptive diagnosis is frequently made prior to all results returning so that treatment may begin, especially in critically ill or deteriorating patients and those with organ failure. Some patients will have a previously known medical condition which is the likely cause of HLH/MAS, such as those with cancer, JIA, or a known genetic cause of recurrent HLH, but most will not. Concurrent testing for underlying causes should be guided by the patient's age, history, and physical exam, as well as the recommendations of pediatric specialists in infectious disease, oncology, and rheumatology. For patients without a clear cause, bone marrow biopsy and

Table 1 Adapted diagnostic criteria for HLH

3 of 4 of the following:
- Fever
- Splenomegaly
- Cytopenia of at least 2 lineages:
    - Hemoglobin <9 g/dL (in infants <4 weeks: hemoglobin <10 g/dL)
    - Platelets $<100 \times 10^9$/L
    - Neutrophils $<1.0 \times 10^9$/L
- Hepatitis

AND 1 of 4 of the following:
- Hemophagocytosis in bone marrow, spleen, liver, or lymph node
- Low or absent natural killer cell activity
- Hyperferritinemia
    - ≥500 μg/L
- High levels of soluble CD25 (soluble interleukin-2 receptor alpha)
    - Age specific

Other results supporting diagnosis:
- Hypertriglyceridemia and/or hypofibrinogenemia
    - Fasting triglycerides 3.0 mmol/L (265 mg/dl)
    - Fibrinogen ≤1.5 g/L

OR

A genetic defect known to be associated with HLH

Note: Because some tests may take a long time to result, some patients may not meet strict diagnostic criteria at the time of treatment initiation

Adapted from Henter et al. [2] and Filipovich [3]

flow cytometry should be completed as soon as possible because HLH-specific therapy includes corticosteroids which can impact the reliability of these tests. Assessment for central nervous system involvement requires lumbar puncture and brain MRI. Other tests for patients without a clear underlying cause typically include bacterial cultures of the blood and urine and often the spinal fluid, viral testing, fungal testing if the patient is immunocompromised, chest X-ray to assess for a mediastinal mass, and antinuclear antibody testing. Patients with encephalitis or significant hepatitis require evaluation for causes of those conditions.

There are a number of conditions on the differential for HLH. With the exception of JIA and MAS, markedly elevated ferritin usually helps differentiate them from HLH. Infection and sepsis are typically the most important acute considerations, and broad antimicrobials should be given until infection is ruled out. Kawasaki disease is another important cause of fever and systemic inflammation in children and can even cause HLH, so HLH should be considered in patients with Kawasaki disease, especially those who do not respond to treatment for Kawasaki disease. Thrombotic thrombocytopenic purpura, hemolytic uremic syndrome, and drug-induced thrombotic microangiopathy are on the differential as they can cause anemia, fever, and renal dysfunction, though evaluation in these conditions reveals a microangiopathic cause of anemia which is not found in HLH. Drug reaction with eosinophilia and systemic symptoms may cause fevers and hepatitis, but does not usually cause the cytopenias typical of HLH. Many causes of encephalitis or hepatitis do not cause the multiorgan dysfunction or markedly elevated ferritin seen in HLH. In patients who have undergone hematopoietic stem cell transfer, transfusion-associated graft-versus-host disease can mimic HLH.

There are many possible complications of HLH depending on the extent of organ damage. Bleeding may occur due to coagulopathy from liver dysfunction or thrombocytopenia. Anemia and thrombocytopenia severe enough to require transfusion are common. Seizures from encephalitis may occur, and hepatitis may lead to encephalopathy. Renal failure requiring dialysis with or without the syndrome of inappropriate antidiuretic hormone sometimes occurs. Respiratory failure, sometimes presenting as acute respiratory distress syndrome, may be severe enough to require intubation. Posterior reversible encephalopathy syndrome can occur, so control of elevated blood pressures is recommended.

Initial management should focus on stabilization of the patient and, if needed, transfer to a facility with the appropriate resources to care for HLH/MAS. Secure intravascular access is vital. Essentially all patients with HLH should initially be given antibiotics until infection is ruled out, and antifungals should be considered in immunosuppressed patients. Patients may require fluid resuscitation and blood products, and patients in shock may require pressors. Hypertension should be managed aggressively. Ideally, corticosteroids are withheld initially until evaluation for oncologic conditions is complete. For patients with an underlying condition causing HLH/MAS, treatment of the underlying condition may be sufficient. HLH-specific therapy is indicated for those with no etiology, with a genetic cause, or who are severely ill. HLH-specific therapy starts with 8 weeks of induction with etoposide and dexamethasone and should be conducted under the supervision of a provider with expertise in doing so [4, 5]. Those with central nervous system involvement typically require intrathecal chemotherapy, usually methotrexate and hydrocortisone. Allogeneic hematopoietic stem cell transfer is frequently performed for patients who do not respond to initial treatment, have certain genetic causes of HLH, or have a hematogenous malignancy. While most patients who survive HLH achieve a normal or near-normal quality of life, long-term neurologic, respiratory, or renal impairment occurs in about 15–20% of survivors. When HLH relapses, it usually does so within 1 year of the initial presentation. The risk of relapse is minimized by avoiding triggers of immune activation and managing underlying conditions.

6 Review Questions

1. Which of the following is the most common trigger of HLH?
   (A) Malignancies
   (B) Rheumatologic conditions
   (C) Fungal infections
   (D) Viral infections
2. Which of the following lab results is NOT suggestive of HLH/MAS?
   (A) Elevated C-reactive protein
   (B) Elevated erythrocyte sedimentation rate
   (C) Elevated ferritin
   (D) Elevated CD25 (soluble interleukin-2 receptor alpha)
3. Which of the following is LEAST likely to be a complication of HLH/MAS?
   (A) Thrombotic microangiopathy
   (B) Posterior reversible encephalopathy syndrome
   (C) Acute respiratory distress syndrome
   (D) Coagulopathy
4. Which of the following is pathognomonic for HLH/MAS?
   (A) Markedly elevated ferritin
   (B) Hepatosplenomegaly
   (C) Hemophagocytosis on bone marrow biopsy
   (D) No finding is pathognomonic for HLH/MAS
5. Which of the following treatment options should ideally be avoided in the initial stabilization of a patient in whom HLH is suspected but who has not yet undergone a diagnostic workup?
   (A) Antibiotics
   (B) Blood products
   (C) Corticosteroids
   (D) Antihypertensives

7 Answers

1. **D**. While all four answer choices can trigger HLH, viral infections are more common than the others.
2. **B**. Despite being a disorder of systemic inflammation, erythrocyte sedimentation rate is often paradoxically low because of the accompanying hypofibrinogenemia.
3. **A**. While the other answer choices are well-documented complications of HLH/MAS, thrombotic microangiopathy would be unexpected. Thrombotic microangiopathy can in some ways mimic HLH/MAS since both may present with anemia and thrombocytopenia, but review of a peripheral blood smear can typically differentiate between these disorders.
4. **D**. Diagnosis of HLH/MAS depends on many factors from the history, physical exam, and laboratory results. Markedly elevated ferritin can occur in systemic JIA without MAS or in patients with iron overload such as those who have received many transfusions. Hepatosplenomegaly is a nonspecific finding of many conditions. Hemophagocytosis on bone marrow biopsy is not always found in HLH/MAS and can be present in other conditions including some malignancies.
5. **C**. HLH/MAS is treated with HLH-specific chemotherapy (often starting with corticosteroids and etoposide), direct treatment of an underlying triggering disorder, hematopoietic stem cell transplant, or some combination of these options. However, corticosteroids should, if possible, not be given until the patient has been evaluated for malignancy since corticosteroids can distort the diagnosis and staging of some malignancies. In the initial stabilization of a patient with HLH, antibiotics are frequently indicated for possible sepsis, blood products are often needed for cytopenias or coagulopathy, and antihypertensives are sometimes necessary to prevent posterior reversible encephalopathy syndrome.

8 Takeaway Points

1. Hemophagocytic lymphohistiocytosis and the related disease macrophage activation syndrome are dangerous disorders of immune hyperactivation affecting multiple organ systems with a high mortality rate.
2. They often present with prolonged fever, hepatosplenomegaly, and a range of lab abnormalities.
3. Triggers include infections, malignancies, immunodeficiencies, immunosuppression, and rheumatologic disorders.
4. Initial stabilization should include secure vascular access, fluid resuscitation, and broad-spectrum antibiotics. Measurement of coagulation factors and chest X-ray to evaluate for a mediastinal mass are indicated. Lumbar puncture and brain MRI should be considered following stabilization.
5. Possible complications of HLH include shock, anemia, bleeding from coagulopathy and thrombocytopenia, encephalopathy, respiratory failure, renal failure, and posterior reversible encephalopathy syndrome.
6. Treatment often involves chemotherapy.

References

1. Jordan MB, Allen CE, Weitzman S, et al. How I treat hemophagocytic lymphohistiocytosis. Blood. 2011;118:4041–52. https://doi.org/10.1182/blood-2011-03-278127.
2. Henter J-I, Horne A, Aricó M, et al. HLH-2004: Diagnostic and therapeutic guidelines for hemophagocytic lymphohistiocytosis. Pediatr Blood Cancer. 2007;48:124–31. https://doi.org/10.1002/pbc.21039.
3. Filipovich AH. Hemophagocytic lymphohistiocytosis (HLH) and related disorders. Hematology. 2009;2009:127–31. https://doi.org/10.1182/asheducation-2009.1.127.
4. Bergsten E, Horne A, Aricó M, et al. Confirmed efficacy of etoposide and dexamethasone in HLH treatment: long-term results of the cooperative HLH-2004 study. Blood. 2017;130:2728–38. https://doi.org/10.1182/blood-2017-06-788349.
5. Henter JI, Aricò M, Egeler RM, et al. HLH-94: a treatment protocol for hemophagocytic lymphohistiocytosis. HLH study Group of the Histiocyte Society. Med Pediatr Oncol. 1997;28:342–7. https://doi.org/10.1002/(sici)1096-911x(199705)28:5<342::aid-mpo3>3.0.co;2-h.

A Child with Medical Complexity and Worsening Irritability

Jonathan Fliegel and Sara Liegel

1 Case Description

A 7-year-old male child with medical complexity (CMC) and severe neurologic impairment presents to the emergency department (ED) with fever, increasing irritability and hypertonia. Over the past 2 days, he has been crying and increasingly fussy, which is unusual for him. A fever today of 104 °C prompted his parents to bring him to the ED. They are concerned about new jittery movements in his arms and legs and that it is now difficult to change his diapers or sit him in his wheelchair because they are unable to relax his hips and knees. Typically, he can drive his own wheelchair, is happy, and communicates nonverbally with squeals and 5–10 signs.

His medical history includes neonatal group B strep (GBS) meningitis leading to hydrocephalus requiring ventriculoperitoneal (VP) shunt placement, neurologic impairment, quadriparetic cerebral palsy with spasticity leading to placement of a baclofen pump, and dysphagia requiring gastrostomy tube feeding. His current scheduled medications include intrathecal baclofen, and polyethylene glycol and senna for constipation.

He has no respiratory symptoms, recent infections, or illness exposures and is tolerating his usual gastrostomy feeds without vomiting or change in daily soft bowel movements. He has never had a seizure.

On exam, he is in moderate distress, diaphoretic, with hypertonic upper and lower extremities. He is febrile (39 °C), tachycardic, and tachypneic. His systolic blood pressure varies between 75 and 100 mm Hg. Notable findings include no rhinorrhea or otitis media, no meningismus, clear lungs, tachycardia with regular rhythm, and a soft abdomen without distention, tenderness, or mass. His arms are

J. Fliegel (✉) · S. Liegel
Department of Pediatrics, University of Wisconsin School of Medicine & Public Health, American Family Children's Hospital, Madison, WI, USA
e-mail: jfliegel@pediatrics.wisc.edu; liegel@pediatrics.wisc.edu

A. Kamzan et al. (eds.), *Children with Medical Complexity in the Emergency Department*, https://doi.org/10.1007/978-3-031-62517-6_8

tightly flexed, legs are extended with scissoring, and he has sustained ankle clonus. He is tremulous with frequent rapid-frequency, low-amplitude movements of his arms and legs that can be suppressed when held. There are no rashes or signs of injury or trauma.

2 Discussion Questions

1. What are leading "not-to-miss" diagnoses?
2. Which labs and studies are urgent initial steps in his evaluation?
3. What are the next best steps in evaluation and management?

3 Case Answers

1. Sepsis, infection, VP shunt malfunction or infection, baclofen withdrawal
2. Assessments for infection and VP shunt malfunction
3. Assessment of baclofen pump, interventions to alleviate baclofen withdrawal

4 Learning Objectives

1. Apply a systematic framework to assess CMC with irritability.
2. Recognize acute autonomic dysfunction (dysautonomia) in CMC.
3. Identify signs of baclofen withdrawal and outline management.

5 Detailed Answer Explanation

This child with medical complexity presents with acute and progressing symptoms of irritability, increased spasticity, hypertonia, atypical movements, and fever. Differential diagnosis in CMC and irritability is broad, and evaluation is challenging. Careful history and physical exam guided by a systematic framework are essential. One framework is GRASP (Guidelines for Ruling out and Assessing Source of Pain) [1]. The most common causes for irritability in these patients are infections or any condition that leads to pain [2]. In addition, like many CMC, he is at risk for complications associated with his medical devices or arising from medication interactions or side effects.

The development of a fever in the context of his irritability should prompt an urgent evaluation for potential infection or sepsis. Initial laboratory assessment may include a complete blood count, inflammatory markers, lactate, urinalysis and urine culture, and blood culture. In this case, several common infections seem less likely based on history and exam, including meningitis, otitis, sinusitis, upper respiratory tract infection, and pneumonia. Similarly with a lack of characteristic symptoms and physical exam findings, several abdominal and musculoskeletal causes of irritability with fever are also less likely. If initial labs are markedly abnormal, or if pertinent signs or symptoms arise, additional labs and imaging may be considered, e.g., serum lipase, metabolic panels, chest radiography, and abdominal or musculoskeletal imaging [1].

Another potential cause that requires urgent evaluation is malfunction or infection of his VP shunt. Cerebrospinal fluid (CSF) shunts are placed most often to alleviate hydrocephalus and drain enlarged ventricles, either into the peritoneum or less often into the right atrium or pleural space. Shunt components include proximal tubing, a valve, reservoir, and distal tubing. Malfunction may occur if a shunt is obstructed or dislodged or if the valve is faulty. Symptoms of CSF shunt malfunction may include irritability, headache, vomiting, changes in behavior or mental status, or seizures [2]. With severe obstruction, patients may manifest with Cushing's triad of bradycardia, hypertension or widened pulse pressure, and irregular respirations, along with other signs of increased intracranial pressure. Patients with distal obstruction may have abdominal pain or show signs of peritonitis. Evaluation of CSF shunt malfunction includes brain imaging with CT or MRI to assess ventricular size and any changes from previous imaging. Radiographs of skull, neck, chest, and abdomen are typically done to assess the position and continuity of the shunt catheter.

In this CMC who has a shunt and fever, the possibility of a CSF shunt infection must also be considered urgently. Though most patients with CSF shunts and fever do not have shunt infections, those who eventually have a shunt infection commonly present with irritability and fever [3]. Shunt infections occur most often within the first few weeks after placement of the shunt, most commonly with skin organisms such as *S. epidermidis*. Infections after the first month and later are less frequent, with enteric organisms being the most common culprits, such as Gram-negative bacilli or anaerobes [3]. If pursued, the evaluation for CSF shunt infection includes obtaining ventricular fluid, typically via a puncture of the shunt reservoir. Pleocytosis, culture, and other diagnostic tests for infection (such as multiplex PCR or 16S rRNA testing) help guide treatment. When concerned about malfunction or infection, early consultation with a neurosurgical specialist is often indicated to assist with assessment, perform a puncture, and, when necessary, remove and replace the shunt.

An alternative diagnosis to consider in this child with a baclofen pump is autonomic dysfunction (dysautonomia) due to withdrawal from intrathecal baclofen (ITB). Withdrawal may occur when baclofen pump tubing is obstructed or dislodged, the reservoir is empty, the pump malfunctions, its battery loses power, or it is removed after an infection. Baclofen has been used for decades to treat spasticity arising from spinal or cerebral causes. It is an agonist for GABA B receptors on pre- and postsynaptic neurons in the central and peripheral nervous system and relaxes spasticity by inhibiting motor neuron activity [4]. Consequently, in cases of baclofen withdrawal syndrome, there is excessive autonomic, neurologic, and psychiatric excitation. Onset of withdrawal symptoms may be rapid, beginning within hours of cessation of baclofen, and they are potentially severe and life-threatening with ITB withdrawal. Initial symptoms may include irritability, tremulousness, pruritus, and paresthesia and can progress to muscle spasms, tremor, myoclonus, increasing spasticity, and muscle rigidity. Fever, tachycardia, and blood pressure changes (more often hypotension) may progress to more severe autonomic instability. Patients can manifest altered mentation with confusion, delirium, hallucinations, or seizures. Rhabdomyolysis may be severe and should be assessed and managed carefully. Progression to multisystem organ failure, cardiac arrest, and death can occur within 1–3 days. These symptoms caused by ITB withdrawal are similar to symptoms in patients with malignant hyperthermia, neuroleptic malignant syndrome, or serotonin syndrome [4].

This child's symptoms of fever, tachycardia, labile blood pressure, myoclonus, and dystonia, along with a change from his baseline mental status, support a diagnosis of baclofen withdrawal syndrome. This requires urgent management. Ideally, baclofen dosing can be restarted expeditiously via the same method. The pump provider, typically a neurosurgery or rehabilitation medicine specialist, must evaluate the pump (reservoir, pump, tubing) and work to resume intrathecal dosing. While awaiting this, enteral baclofen and intravenous benzodiazepines are the mainstays of treatment and may be titrated to alleviate symptoms. Other options have been used successfully, including cyproheptadine (first-line), propofol, dantrolene, and dexmedetomidine [4]. Patients with baclofen withdrawal syndrome may require management in an intensive care unit to monitor for respiratory depression after high doses of benzodiazepines or these alternative medications and for management of potential complications including autonomic instability, multisystem organ failure, and severe rhabdomyolysis.

Children with medical complexity may also present with symptoms of autonomic dysfunction (dysautonomia) in other settings. Chronic symptoms such as hypothermia, cool extremities, ileus, or irregular respiratory drive may be related to abnormal regulation by areas of the hypothalamus, medulla, and pons that control these autonomic functions [2]. Alternatively, episodes of sympathetic hyperactivity may occur sporadically in CMC, which may be evaluated using a systematic framework such as GRASP, as noted above [1]. A specific version of dysautonomia has been defined as paroxysmal sympathetic hyperactivity (PSH), which can occur in children and adults after severe acute brain injuries, such as traumatic brain injury, stroke, hypoxic-ischemic encephalopathy, or CNS infection [2]. Symptoms of PSH include tachycardia, tachypnea, hypertension, hyperthermia, and dystonia. Scoring systems for PSH are helpful for diagnosis, assessing severity, and monitoring interventions. Treatment of PSH typically includes medications for sympathetic excess (beta-blockers, clonidine) and pain (opiates, gabapentin).

6 Review Questions

1. A 10-year-old child with neurologic impairment, hydrocephalus, ventriculoperitoneal (VP) shunt placed 9 years ago, spasticity, and baclofen pump presents to an ED for increased lethargy. He has had rhinorrhea and cough for 2–3 days, and a rapid viral test was positive for influenza yesterday. On exam, vital signs include a temperature of 37.5 °C, heart rate of 45 beats/min, respirations of 10 per minute with irregular pauses, and blood pressure of 140/90 mm Hg. He is somnolent and arouses only with sternal rub.

   Of the following, the most likely diagnosis is:

   (A) Baclofen withdrawal syndrome
   (B) Sepsis
   (C) VP shunt malfunction
   (D) VP shunt infection

2. A 4-year-old child had a baclofen pump placed recently. Her parents are pleased that his spasticity is improved but are concerned that she is weak, seems limp, and feels cool to the touch with a temperature of 35.5 ° C. They also say that she is seeing bananas floating in her room.

   Of the following, symptoms that help distinguish between baclofen toxicity and withdrawal include all of the following EXCEPT:

   (A) Hallucinations
   (B) Hypothermia
   (C) Hypotonia
   (D) Somnolence

3. An 8-year-old boy has a history of cerebral palsy and spasticity. He presents to the ED with a fever of 38.5 °C, increased muscle tone and reflexes, and confusion. His parents are separated, and the child just returned from visiting his father for 2 weeks. He has missed doses of baclofen for the past several days. He is given a dose of his oral baclofen.

   Of the following, a first-line medication to improve his overall symptoms is (a):
   (A) Nonsteroidal anti-inflammatory drug (NSAID)
   (B) Botulinum-A injection
   (C) Benzodiazepine
   (D) Propofol

7 Answers

1. **C.** The patient's vital sign abnormalities fit Cushing's triad of bradycardia, hypertension, and irregular respirations, and his mental status is depressed. These are signs of increased intracranial pressure, most likely occurring due to

VP shunt malfunction. Patients with baclofen withdrawal syndrome have excessive excitation, with tachycardia and hypotension more often than hypertension, myoclonus, and hypertonia. Those with sepsis may be lethargic but typically have tachycardia and hypotension. A minority of VP shunt malfunctions (3–8%) are caused by infection, and infections are much less frequent beyond the first few months after placement.

2. **A.** Certain symptoms differ between baclofen toxicity and withdrawal. Toxicity may occur if dosing is too high. This risk is higher with intrathecal dosing, although toxicity may occur with enteral dosing. Symptoms that occur with baclofen toxicity include hypothermia, hypotonia, hyporeflexia, and somnolence (excess inhibitory effects), while symptoms with baclofen withdrawal include hyperthermia, hypertonia, hyperreflexia, and anxiety (excess excitatory effects). Hallucinations may occur in either. Heart rate and blood pressure do not distinguish between these conditions, since bradycardia or tachycardia and hypotension or hypertension may occur in either. Baclofen withdrawal is more severe, with possible rhabdomyolysis, which does not occur with baclofen toxicity.
3. **C.** Chronic baclofen use leads to downregulation of GABA B receptors. Cessation of baclofen leads to hyperactivity of afferent nerves, resulting in the symptoms of baclofen withdrawal. Resuming baclofen is the first step to treat withdrawal. Medications that enhance GAB A-mediated synaptic inhibition are used to alleviate withdrawal symptoms. Benzodiazepines do this by action through GABA A receptors and are considered first-line adjuncts. Propofol works similarly and may be used second line in more severe cases. NSAIDs treat fever, and botulinum-A injections are used to alleviate focal spasticity, but neither address the underlying mechanism in baclofen withdrawal.

8 Takeaway Points

1. Since the differential diagnosis for irritability and pain in children with medical complexity is broad, using a systematic approach is essential.
2. Symptoms of abrupt intrathecal baclofen (ITB) withdrawal may include fever and increased spasticity and can progress to hallucinations, delirium, seizures, and muscle rigidity and potentially to severe autonomic instability, rhabdomyolysis, cardiac arrest, and even death.
3. The symptoms of severe baclofen withdrawal syndrome are similar to symptoms seen in patients with sepsis, malignant hyperthermia, neuroleptic malignant syndrome, serotonin syndrome, and paroxysmal sympathetic hyperactivity (PSH).
4. The primary treatment for baclofen withdrawal is resumption of baclofen dosing. Management options include benzodiazepines and cyproheptadine (first-line), propofol, dantrolene, and dexmedetomidine.

5. Patients with baclofen withdrawal syndrome may require management in an intensive care unit for respiratory depression, autonomic instability, or severe rhabdomyolysis.
6. Symptoms of autonomic dysfunction (dysautonomia) may also be present in patients with paroxysmal sympathetic hyperactivity (PSH) and sporadically or chronically in children with medical complexity.

References

1. Morse BL, Solodiuk JC, Greco CD, et al. Initial validation of GRASP: a differential diagnoses algorithm for children with medical complexity and an unknown source of pain. Hosp Pediatr. 2020;10(8):633–40.
2. Hall DE, Glader L, Mauskar S. Acute care of the child with medical complexity. In: Zaoutis LB, Chiang VW, editors. Comprehensive pediatric hospital medicine. 2nd ed. New York: McGraw-Hill Education; 2018. p. 983–7.
3. McCulloh R, Thomson J. Device related infections. In: Zaoutis LB, Chiang VW, editors. Comprehensive pediatric hospital medicine. 2nd ed. New York: McGraw-Hill Education; 2018. p. 585–9.
4. Romito JW, Turner ER, Rosener JA, et al. Baclofen therapeutics, toxicity, and withdrawal: a narrative review. SAGE Open Med. 2021;9:1–13.

Cystic Fibrosis Pulmonary Exacerbation

Harrison Luttrell, Jeffrey C. Winer, and Tonia E. Gardner

1 Case

A 12-year-old African American female with cystic fibrosis (CF) presents to the emergency department (ED) with worsening productive cough and chest pain. She follows closely with her pulmonologist in a care center several hours from her hometown and your emergency department. She had been in her usual state of health until 7 days prior to presentation, when she developed a nonproductive cough and rhinorrhea after her sister had similar symptoms. At that time, she was prescribed oral antibiotics and increased her airway clearance regimen from twice daily to four times daily, but she has had continued worsening of her symptoms.

She has a history of recurrent pulmonary exacerbations that have required admission for intravenous (IV) antibiotics, with the most recent being about 3 months previously. After her most recent admission, her forced expiratory volume in one second (FEV1) improved to her baseline of 90% predicted. Her parents usually take her directly to the care center. However, this time they noticed that her sputum had streaks of blood and were worried about the onset of chest pain, which she has not had with previous exacerbations. They reached out to her primary pulmonologist who suggested they be evaluated quickly. As a result, they made the decision to take her directly to the closest ED.

On presentation to the ED, she appears fatigued but is breathing comfortably in room air with an oxygen saturation of 97%. Her lung exam is notable for diffuse

H. Luttrell (✉)
Department of Medicine, Vanderbilt University Medical Center, Nashville, TN, USA
e-mail: harrison.luttrell@vumc.org

J. C. Winer · T. E. Gardner
Department of Pediatrics, Le Bonheur Children's Hospital, University of Tennessee Health Science Center, Memphis, TN, USA
e-mail: jwiner1@uthsc.edu; tgardn13@uthsc.edu

A. Kamzan et al. (eds.), *Children with Medical Complexity in the Emergency Department*, https://doi.org/10.1007/978-3-031-62517-6_9

inspiratory fine crackles bilaterally, which are worst in the left lower lung fields. During your examination, she has intermittent coughing fits and produces greenish sputum with a small streak of blood in it.

2 Discussion Questions

1. What complication of cystic fibrosis is this patient most likely experiencing?
2. What is the next best step in evaluation and management?

3 Case Answers

1. The above case is of a child with known cystic fibrosis (CF) and presenting with progressive cough and chest pain. These symptoms are hallmarks of a CF pulmonary exacerbation.
2. Because a common complication of CF is pneumothorax, early evaluation with a chest X-ray is important to rule this out before providing respiratory treatments that could exacerbate a pneumothorax. While the patient has scant hemoptysis, this is common in CF pulmonary exacerbations and is not itself an additional concern.

4 Learning Objectives

1. Describe the pathophysiology of CF.
2. Recognize and identify common complications of CF pulmonary exacerbations.
3. Describe the initial management of a patient presenting to a community ED with a CF pulmonary exacerbation.
4. Recognize the limitations of current modulator therapy for CF patients.

5 Discussion

CF is a rare genetic disease that is regularly encountered by practitioners who care for pediatric patients. CF as a disease process is more common in individuals of Indo-European descent, though it is still prevalent in those of Hispanic, African, and Asian descent. CF is an autosomal recessive condition resulting from mutations in the *CFTR* gene on chromosome 7q31.2 [1]. This gene codes for the cystic fibrosis transmembrane conductance regulator (CFTR), which is expressed in cells throughout multiple organs in the body. CFTR functions as a chloride channel on the surface of cells to hydrate secretions, and its absence leads to the formation of thick secretions and mucus. There are numerous genetic mutations (>2000 variants) that affect the way this channel is transported to the cell surface or functions [1]. The most common mutation is known as *F508del* in which the CFTR protein is made but is unable to be transported to the cell surface due to misfolding [1]. Due to CFTR expression in multiple organs, CF disease manifests with pulmonary, gastrointestinal, reproductive, and endocrine pathology. As of 2010, all states in the United States have mandatory CF screening with immunoreactive trypsinogen, and some will perform follow-up confirmatory testing as well. Since the advent of newborn screening, most patients with CF are diagnosed as infants by a confirmatory pilocarpine sweat test after a positive test on newborn screen testing.

In the lung, inappropriate CFTR function results in the development of inspissated secretions that cause mucus plugging. This mucus plugging results in inflammation and predisposition to infection, which leads to progressive decline in lung function over time. In addition to this chronic decline in lung function, patients with CF often have periods of acute worsening in their symptoms and lung function, which are known as pulmonary exacerbations. During exacerbations, patients often report pulmonary symptoms including wheezing, cough, and sputum production [1]. Although CF patients often present directly to CF care centers in pulmonary exacerbations, there are times, such as in our case, that patients may present to the local ED for initial stabilization.

Airway clearance therapy (ACT) is an essential component of maintenance therapy in patients with CF and in those with pulmonary exacerbations. Individuals with CF have an ACT regimen that is personalized to their age, patient preferences, and severity of illness. Some of the more common methods include oscillatory positive expiratory pressure, manual percussion and postural drainage, and high-frequency chest compression, often with vest therapy. These therapies are often administered in conjunction with aerosolized albuterol, recombinant human (rh) DNase (dornase alfa/Pulmozyme), and hypertonic saline. Recommendations suggest patients undergo ACT at least twice daily even when well [1]. However, in the setting of a pulmonary exacerbation, active infection and decreased mucus clearance necessitate more frequent and longer sessions of airway clearance [2]. It is not uncommon for patients to receive therapy as frequently as every 4 hours while undergoing treatment for pulmonary exacerbation. In the acute setting, performing ACT on patients with pulmonary exacerbation may help with symptoms while awaiting further advice from the patient's CF care center.

Treatment for pulmonary exacerbations involves the use of antibiotic therapy in addition to increased ACT as above. Infectious pathogens play an important role in the pathophysiology of CF and pulmonary exacerbations. As a result of increased thickness of secretions and decreased mucociliary clearance, bacterial overgrowth occurs and leads to inflammation and destruction of lung tissue. Pathogens associated with this bacterial overgrowth in CF are different than the typical pathogens associated with community-acquired pneumonia in otherwise healthy patients. The two most noteworthy pathogens include *Pseudomonas aeruginosa* and

Staphylococcus aureus. Individual patients have a unique culture history that often evolves over time. Antibiotic therapy is guided based on prior sputum culture results and resistance patterns. Therapy decisions that address chronic suppression and treatment of acute pulmonary exacerbations are often made by multidisciplinary teams that include pulmonologists and pharmacists at CF care centers. Although antibiotic choice and therapy play an essential role in the treatment of pulmonary exacerbations, there is no evidence to suggest that urgent administration of intravenous antibiotics improves outcomes. As a result, it is appropriate to wait for further recommendations from a patient's CF care center prior to initiating antibiotics in most cases. It is important to note that sputum cultures in patients with CF require unique care and attention. Microbiology labs in CF care centers pay particular attention to CF sputum cultures and specifically look for organisms that are uniquely found in patients with CF, such as *P. aeruginosa* and *S. aureus*. As a result, collecting sputum cultures at a facility that is not familiar with the care of CF patients may produce results of limited utility.

Although generally a non-emergent condition, some potentially life-threatening complications of CF are important to rule out and be conscious of during initial workup. These include hemoptysis and pneumothorax. Hemoptysis is a known, potentially life-threatening complication of CF and can occur during pulmonary exacerbations and in patients with severe lung disease. Management of hemoptysis largely depends on the volume of blood produced. Guidelines classify hemoptysis as scant if less than 5 milliliters (mL), mild-to-moderate if between 5 and 240 mL, and massive if over 240 mL [3]. Most cases of hemoptysis in patients with CF self-resolve. However, patients who present with massive hemoptysis and are clinically unstable despite resuscitation may require urgent intervention. The intervention of choice in that case is bronchial artery embolization and should be pursued prior to any additional studies (e.g., bronchoscopy, computed tomography of the chest) [3]. Importantly, both aerosol therapies and airway clearance should be withheld in patients with massive hemoptysis. However, they can be safely continued in patients with scant hemoptysis. Recommendations are not made about appropriate therapies for patients with mild-moderate hemoptysis, which again emphasizes the need for early involvement of practitioners familiar with the complications of CF. Importantly, presence of scant or mild-to-moderate hemoptysis without other symptoms of pulmonary exacerbation necessitates treatment with antibiotic therapy [3].

Another potential complication of CF lung disease is the development of pneumothorax. Pneumothoraxes are defined by their size, with small being less than or equal to 3 centimeters (cm) from the apex to the cupola and large being greater than 3 cm. A chest tube is indicated for CF patients with a large pneumothorax or clinical instability [3]. In patients with a pneumothorax, intrapulmonary percussive ventilation, high-frequency chest compression, and positive expiratory pressure ACT should be withheld for at least 2 weeks [1].

In recent years, CFTR modulators have had dramatic effects on the lung function of individuals with CF. There are several CFTR modulators that are currently in use: ivacaftor (Kalydeco), lumacaftor/ivacaftor (Orkambi), tezacaftor/ivacaftor

(Symdeko), and elexacaftor/tezacaftor/ivacaftor (Trikafta). Each of these CF modulators has a different mechanism of action that either allows for increased function of existing CFTR proteins or allows more protein to be expressed on the cell surface [1]. Although these medications have been shown to improve pulmonary function, each medication is limited for use in patients with specific mutations, often *F508del*, and to patients of certain ages. For example, Trikafta has shown significant improvement in multiple signs of disease but is only approved for patients over 2 years of age and who have at least one *F508del* mutation. Although many patients qualify for modulator therapy, there are still those who are either limited by age or who have rare mutations that cannot receive therapy at this time. As a result, it is important that we continue to educate providers on how to manage CF pulmonary exacerbations and acute emergencies as they are likely to continue to be issues for years to come.

6 Review Questions

1. A 7-year-old patient was recently diagnosed with cystic fibrosis in the setting of chronic pancreatitis and frequent pneumonias. Neonatal state screening was negative at birth including for cystic fibrosis. They had an abnormal pilocarpine sweat test but have not yet seen a pulmonologist. On examination, they are well-appearing, but have signs of moderate malnourishment. Of the following, the diagnostic test that could determine their eligibility for a CFTR modulator is:

   (A) CFTR gene sequencing
   (B) Fecal pancreatic elastase
   (C) Immunoreactive trypsinogen
   (D) Pulmonary function testing

2. A 15-year-old patient with cystic fibrosis is admitted to a community hospital for multifocal pneumonia. The patient is well-appearing other than moderate tachypnea and respiratory distress. No previous records are available for the patient because the family just moved from another state. Of the following, the patient's cystic fibrosis puts them at the biggest increased risk of infection by which organism?

   (A) Influenza A virus
   (B) Nontypeable *Haemophilus influenzae*
   (C) *Pseudomonas aeruginosa*
   (D) *Streptococcus pneumoniae*

3. A 14-year-old patient with cystic fibrosis presents to the hospital due to bloody sputum. They awoke this morning with worsening violent coughing and found a small streak of blood on one of the tissues. The event occurred approximately

60 min ago, and there has been no further bleeding. Of the following, the most appropriate next step for this hemoptysis is to:

(A) Arrange for urgent transfer for bronchoscopy
(B) Begin airway clearance therapy
(C) Obtain complete blood count
(D) Perform bronchial artery embolization

7 Answers

1. **A.** CFTR gene sequencing. This patient has an increased likelihood of having a rare cystic fibrosis mutation as the cause of their disease due to the normal newborn screening and relatively mild symptoms. CFTR gene sequencing will determine the patient's mutation(s) and eligibility for CFTR modulators.
2. **C.** *Pseudomonas aeruginosa*. Patients with cystic fibrosis are at particularly high risk of infection and colonization from *Pseudomonas aeruginosa* and *Staphylococcus aureus* (including methicillin-resistant species). As a result, empiric antibiotic treatment should generally include coverage for these pathogens, such as an aminoglycoside or fourth-generation cephalosporin for *P. aeruginosa* and vancomycin for methicillin-resistant *S. aureus*. For patients with cystic fibrosis, it is usually better to tailor their initial antibiotics to their previous culture results, if available. Additionally, if available, respiratory cultures should be performed at specific microbiology laboratories due to differences in protocol from other respiratory cultures.
3. **B.** Begin airway clearance therapy. In this case, the patient has scant, self-resolved hemoptysis. This is a very common symptom in the setting of cystic fibrosis exacerbation and does not necessitate additional workup or intervention. Although patients with massive bleeding should have airway clearance therapy held until the bleeding is stopped, airway clearance therapy is safe in patients with scant hemoptysis.

8 Takeaway Points

1. CF is an autosomal recessive condition caused by mutations in the CFTR gene, which leads to thickened secretions resulting in damage to multiple organ systems.
2. Coordination with CF care centers is essential for the appropriate management of patients with manifestations of CF, including pulmonary exacerbations.
3. Massive hemoptysis and pneumothorax are life-threatening complications of CF and should be ruled out and managed emergently if present.

4. ACTs are essential components of the acute and maintenance care of patients with CF but should be held in certain circumstances, such as massive hemoptysis and pneumothorax.
5. CFTR modulator therapies are effective in improving measures of disease severity in patients with CF but are limited to specific populations and genetic mutations.

References

1. Dickinson KM, Collaco JM. Cystic fibrosis. Pediatr Rev. 2021;42(2):55–67.
2. Flume PA, et al. Cystic fibrosis pulmonary guidelines: treatment of pulmonary exacerbations. Am J Respir Crit Care Med. 2009;180(9):802–8.
3. Flume PA, et al. Cystic fibrosis pulmonary guidelines: pulmonary complications: hemoptysis and pneumothorax. Am J Respir Crit Care Med. 2010;182(3):298–306.

An Infant Born at Extreme Prematurity Presenting in Respiratory Distress

Alexandra Vinci, Dimpy Mody, Tuan Nguyen, and Thomas Duggan

1 Case

A 3.5-month-old male infant born at 24 + 3 weeks gestation, now corrected to 39 + 1 weeks, is brought to the emergency department (ED) by his mother with a chief complaint of "breathing fast." Per mother's report, the infant has been ill for approximately 12 h with irritability, crying, decreased interest in feeding, clear rhinorrhea, and a temperature of 100.7 °F. His symptoms have been worsening over the last 4 h, reported as "faster breathing with his ribs showing." His 3-year-old sister attends daycare and has cough and congestion with positive rapid assay for respiratory syncytial virus at the pediatrician's office.

The patient's medical history includes the following neonatal intensive care unit (NICU) course: preterm delivery due to severe maternal preeclampsia, respiratory distress syndrome that required high-frequency ventilation and surfactant therapy, moderate bronchopulmonary dysplasia, pulmonary hypertension treated with inhaled nitric oxide (iNO), apnea of prematurity treated with caffeine, anemia of prematurity requiring multiple packed red blood cell transfusions, hyperbilirubinemia requiring 7 days of phototherapy, hypoglycemia, persistent feeding intolerance, bilateral grade 2 intraventricular hemorrhage, and retinopathy of prematurity.

His vital signs in the ED are as follows: heart rate 155 bpm, respiratory rate 72 breaths/min, blood pressure 89/42, and oxygen saturation 86% in room air.

On physical exam, the baby exhibits intercostal and suprasternal retractions, nasal flaring, expiratory grunting, and head bobbing. Breath sounds are coarse with diffuse rales. His mucous membranes are tacky. A grade 3 systolic murmur with

A. Vinci (✉) · D. Mody · T. Nguyen · T. Duggan
NYU Grossman School of Medicine, New York, NY, USA
e-mail: alexandra.vinci@nyulangone.org; Dimpy.Mody@nyulangone.org; Tuan.Nguyen@nyulangone.org; Thomas.Duggan@nyulangone.org

A. Kamzan et al. (eds.), *Children with Medical Complexity in the Emergency Department*, https://doi.org/10.1007/978-3-031-62517-6_10

loud S2 is heard on cardiac auscultation. His abdomen is soft, non-tender, and non-distended with no palpable masses. His pulses are 1+ and thready with capillary refill time of 4 s.

2 Discussion Questions

1. What is the next best step in management?
2. What complications should be anticipated as a result of the underlying diagnosis and/or from the treatment?

3 Case Answers

1. This infant, born extremely premature with a history of bronchopulmonary dysplasia (BPD), chronic lung disease (CLD), and persistent pulmonary hypertension (PPHN), is presenting to the emergency department in acute hypoxic respiratory failure likely due to bronchiolitis. The next best step in management is to initiate respiratory support with high-flow nasal cannula. In addition, hydration status should be improved with intravenous fluids, however with caution given the patient's underlying PPHN.
2. Apnea, pulmonary hypertension crisis, and pneumothorax are potential complications. These would dictate a more thorough and aggressive diagnostic evaluation and interventions including chest radiography, cardiac evaluation, and pharmacologic therapies.

4 Learning Objectives

1. Review the effect of extreme prematurity on lung parenchyma that includes development of bronchopulmonary dysplasia and increased lifetime risk of respiratory illness.
2. Discuss bronchiolitis and the acute management of respiratory failure in patients born at extreme prematurity with chronic lung disease including various modes of respiratory support, medications, nutritional support, and fluid resuscitation.
3. Discuss pulmonary hypertension pathophysiology and pulmonary hypertensive crisis management.
4. Review the criteria for palivizumab RSV prophylaxis.

5 Discussion

5.1 Bronchopulmonary Dysplasia

Bronchopulmonary dysplasia is a chronic lung disease that primarily affects preterm infants who require mechanical ventilation or oxygen supplementation in the NICU [1]. BPD is one of the most common complications of preterm birth, affecting approximately 10,000 infants in the United States each year. It is characterized by inflammation, injury, and abnormal development of the pulmonary architecture and vasculature leading to impaired gas exchange, airway obstruction, and persistent respiratory symptoms [2]. BPD has a significant impact on long-term morbidity and mortality and is a cause of increased healthcare resources and costs [3].

The pathophysiology of BPD is multifactorial, involving environmental and genetic factors that interact to disrupt normal lung development and function [4–6]. Premature birth hinders lung development prior to normal surfactant production, causing respiratory distress syndrome (RDS) and impaired gas exchange [6, 7]. Disordered alveolar growth and pulmonary vascular development, coupled with postnatal exposure to oxygen, lead to inflammation and lung injury [5]. Mechanical ventilation and oxygen supplementation are often necessary to support the respiratory function of preterm infants; however, these therapies exacerbate oxidative stress, lung injury, and BPD [8]. This further promotes abnormal repair and remod eling of lung tissue and vasculature, resulting in fibrosis, smooth muscle hyperplasia, and simplified alveolar architecture. Physiologically, BPD causes reduced lung function and abnormal gas exchange [8].

Overall, BPD severity and phenotype variability involve the interplay between many complex mechanisms for injury, including gestational age, arrested pulmonary and vascular development, inflammation, infection, oxidative stress, nutrition, and genetics [5]. The diagnosis of mild, moderate, or severe BPD is based on a combination of clinical, radiological, and physiological criteria, according to the consensus definition of the National Institutes of Health workshop on BPD summarized in Table 1 [9].

Table 1 Summary of the diagnostic criteria for BPD

		Gestational age at birth <32 weeks: Evaluate at 36-week postmenstrual age or discharge, whichever comes first	**Gestational age at birth ≥32 weeks:** Evaluate at >28 days but <56 days postnatal age or discharge, whichever comes first
Mild	Required treatment with FiO_2 >0.21 for at least 28 days plus:	Room air	Room air
Moderate		Need for FiO_2 <0.3	Need for FiO_2 <0.3
Severe		Need for FiO_2 >0.3 and/or positive pressure[a]	Need for FiO_2 >0.3 and/or positive pressure[a]

[a]Includes positive-pressure ventilation or nasal continuous positive airway pressure

The primary mechanism for BPD reduction is prevention. Current strategies include antenatal corticosteroids, surfactant administration, noninvasive ventilation, vitamin A, caffeine, and optimal nutritional support [10]. Diuretics, bronchodilators, postnatal corticosteroids, patent ductus arteriosus closure, and fluid restriction are commonly employed but remain controversial due to adverse effect profiles and conflicting evidence [10]. Noninvasive respiratory support with CPAP or HFNC is preferred over invasive mechanical ventilation whenever possible [11]. Oxygen supplementation should be titrated to achieve adequate oxygen saturation while avoiding hyperoxia, which worsens oxidative stress and lung injury [12]. Early initiation of enteral feeding with adequate calories and protein remains crucial for optimal growth and development [12].

BPD is associated with complications that include chronic respiratory insufficiency, infection, and neurodevelopmental impairment [13–15]. Respiratory complications of BPD include increased airway resistance, reduced lung compliance, and air trapping, resulting in recurrent respiratory infections and exacerbations [13, 14]. BPD causes an increased risk of developing pulmonary hypertension—a potentially fatal condition characterized by elevated blood pressure in the pulmonary circulation, leading to right ventricular failure [13]. The baby in this vignette, having already had a history of pulmonary hypertension, is at high risk for this very serious complication.

5.2 *Acute Bronchiolitis*

Bronchiolitis is the leading cause of lower respiratory tract infections and pediatric hospitalizations for patients under 2 years of age [16]. Bronchiolitis may be triggered by any respiratory virus; however, RSV is a leading cause [16]. Symptoms typically begin with cough, rhinorrhea, congestion, and fever before progressing to increased work of breathing, feeding difficulties, and, in severe cases, respiratory failure and the need for mechanical ventilation [17]. Criteria for hospital admission include oxygen saturation <92% on room air, decreased feeding volumes of ~50% of normal, dehydration, apnea, and significant respiratory distress (i.e., grunting, nasal flaring, respiratory rate >70 breaths/min, severe use of chest wall muscles) [18].

Infants born prematurely with a history of chronic lung disease, congenital heart lesions, Trisomy 21, and/or neuromuscular disease are at high risk of apneic episodes, severe disease, and need for aggressive respiratory support [16]. The baby in this case is particularly vulnerable given their extensive clinical course in the NICU that includes bronchopulmonary dysplasia, chronic lung disease, and persistent pulmonary hypertension.

Supportive care with supplemental oxygen, intravenous hydration, reestablishing enteral feeds, and close clinical monitoring remain the mainstays of treatment, regardless of the gestational age at birth and postnatal course [16, 17]. Feeds may be attempted orally but transitioned to nasogastric if work of breathing hinders appropriate feeding coordination [16–18]. Oxygen via simple nasal cannula is typically the initial step to improve oxygenation. High-flow nasal cannula (HFNC) noninvasively delivers high levels of heated and humidified oxygen without damaging respiratory endothelium and may reduce transfers to pediatric intensive care and the need for invasive forms of oxygenation [16]. Flow is usually started at 1–2 L/kg. Continuous positive airway pressure (CPAP) and bi-level positive airway pressure (BiPAP) may be utilized if noninvasive means of oxygenation are unsuccessful [16]. Mechanical ventilation should be reserved for patients in persistent respiratory failure despite other modes of oxygenation [16].

Bronchodilators are not recommended with bronchiolitis except when there is a history of atopy [16, 18]. A one-time administration of albuterol may be trialed to assess response [16]. Glucocorticoids, racemic epinephrine, heliox, and leukotriene inhibitors are not routinely recommended [16, 18]. Chest physiotherapy does not improve disease severity or decrease length of stay (LOS) but may be employed in patients with impaired airway clearance [16, 18]. Nebulized hypertonic saline improves mucociliary clearance and has been shown to potentially decrease LOS in some studies [16–18]. Chest radiography often shows respiratory infiltrates from atelectasis indistinguishable from bacterial infection and may lead to overtreatment; hence, they are not routinely recommended unless there is suspicion for bacterial pneumonia [19]. Antibiotics are only recommended for patients with bacterial infection [16–18].

5.3 *Pulmonary Hypertensive Crisis*

Emergency medicine providers must consider pulmonary hypertensive crisis (PHC) in any infant with a history of prematurity and PPHN presenting with respiratory distress, hypoxemia, and signs of impending cardiogenic shock. This baby is at high risk for developing PHC given his past medical history.

After birth, PPHN is due to failure of transitioning from fetal circulation to normal extrauterine circulation. Its incidence is approximately 2 per 1000 live births in the United States [20]. Risk factors include prematurity and birth weight small or large for gestational age in addition to perinatal exposure to selective serotonin reuptake inhibitors, nonsteroidal anti-inflammatory drugs, maternal smoking, maternal diabetes, and maternal obesity [21].

The physiological cardiopulmonary transition of the newborn involves two main mechanisms: an increase in systemic arterial pressure and a reduction of pulmonary vascular resistance (PVR). During fetal development, the placenta is the essential organ of gas exchange. Prenatally, right ventricular output is diverted away from the fluid-filled lungs and crosses the foramen ovale and the ductus arteriosus to the aorta, known as right-to-left shunting. Shortly after birth, umbilical cord clamping removes the low-resistance placental circulation leading to the increase in systemic arterial pressure [22]. The first postnatal breath provides lung aeration and distention with increased alveolar oxygen tension and production of vasodilatory factors such as nitric oxide and prostacyclin from pulmonary endothelium, decreasing PVR and increasing pulmonary blood flow [23]. This closes the foramen ovale, and blood flow reverses across the ductus arteriosus and subsequently closes the ductus arteriosus and ductus venosus, resulting in equalized left and right ventricular function in the normal newborn [24].

Disruption of these mechanisms leads to the multifactorial pathogenesis of persistent pulmonary hypertension of the newborn. Etiologies include lung parenchymal diseases such as meconium aspiration syndrome, neonatal pneumonia, sepsis, and, as in this baby's case, respiratory distress syndrome and bronchopulmonary dysplasia—particularly in neonates who require mechanical ventilation. Increased pulmonary arteriolar vasoconstriction and vascular structural remodeling increase PVR, leading to persistence of right-to-left shunting [25].

Immediate assessment with a thorough history and physical in an infant with a history of pulmonary hypertension is vital in the emergency room. This baby's physical exam is notable for a loud murmur and signs of cardiogenic shock (weak pulses and delayed capillary refill time). In addition to establishing adequate oxygenation, initial diagnostic evaluation includes electrocardiogram, chest radiograph, echocardiogram, and consultation with a pediatric cardiologist. If pulmonary hypertensive crisis is confirmed, transfer to a center with pediatric pulmonary hypertension experience should be considered [26, 27].

While awaiting transfer, goals of therapy encompass minimizing metabolic and hypoxic stress, optimizing ventilation, careful fluid resuscitation in small aliquots of 5–10 mL/kg to avoid worsening right ventricular dysfunction, and pulmonary vasodilator therapy [28]. Pharmacologic options for pulmonary hypertension are summarized in Table 2 [29].

Table 2 Pharmacologic therapy for pediatric pulmonary hypertension

Drug	Drug class	Dosing	Potential adverse effects
Inhaled nitric oxide	Exogenous nitric oxide	Starting dose: 20 ppm, inhaled	Methemoglobinemia, airway irritation
Sildenafil	Phosphodiesterase inhibitor (PDE5)	Age <12 months: 0.5 mg/kg three times daily, orally Weight <20 kg: 10 mg three times daily, orally Weight >20 kg: 10 mg three times daily, orally	Headache, nasal congestion, flushing, hypotension, agitation, priapism Avoid nitrates
Epoprostenol	Prostacyclin (PGI2)	Starting dose: 1–2 ng/kg/min, continuous intravenous infusion Maintenance dose: 50–80 ng/kg/min	Headache, flushing, diarrhea, jaw, foot and bone pain, thrombocytopenia, hypotension

(continued)

Table 2 (continued)

Drug	Drug class	Dosing	Potential adverse effects
Treprostinil	Prostacyclin (PGI2)	Starting dose: 1–2 ng/kg/min, continuous intravenous or subcutaneous infusion	Headache, flushing, diarrhea, muscle pain, pain at subcutaneous injection site
Iloprost	Prostacyclin (PGI2)	Starting dose: 2.5 mcg 6 times per day, inhaled Maintenance dose: 5 mcg 6–9 times per day, inhaled	Headaches, flushing, cough, wheeze, jaw pain, diarrhea, hypotension at higher doses
Bosentan	Endothelin receptor antagonist (ET_A and ET_B dual antagonist)	Starting dose is one-half the maintenance dose Maintenance dose: Weight <10 kg: 2 mg/kg twice daily, orally Weight 10–20 kg: 31.25 mg twice daily, orally Weight 20–40 kg: 62.5 mg twice daily, orally Weight >40 kg: 125 mg twice daily, orally	Headache, nasal congestion, flushing, abdominal pain, vomiting, risk for hepatotoxicity, fluid retention, concurrent use with sildenafil may increase bosentan serum levels and decrease sildenafil serum levels

5.4 Pneumothorax

The baby's baseline chronic lung disease, coupled with the potential for cardiopulmonary resuscitation and need for mechanical ventilation during acute management, places him at increased risk for pneumothorax. A pneumothorax, or air between visceral and parietal pleura, arises from air leak through breaks in lung tissue [30]. Pneumothorax may also exist on initial presentation prior to any medical interventions, complicating the clinical picture of the patient. Emergency medicine providers should maintain a high index of suspicion for pneumothoraces for any infant in respiratory distress but especially when there is a history of chronic lung disease and prematurity. Pneumothorax is classified as follows [30, 31]:

Spontaneous	Traumatic
Primary: no known lung conditions	Accidental: penetrating or blunt trauma
Secondary: underlying acute or chronic lung disease, like bronchopulmonary dysplasia, asthma, cystic fibrosis, respiratory distress syndrome, and meconium aspiration syndrome	Iatrogenic: mechanical or positive-pressure ventilation, central line placement, thoracentesis or bronchoscopy

Mechanical ventilation with high tidal volumes and high peak pressures increases the risk for barotrauma and pneumothorax [32, 33]. This further supports the notion that noninvasive oxygenation via HFNC and/or BiPAP should be used whenever possible.

Physical exam in infants with pneumothorax shows decreased breath sounds, decreased chest excursion on the affected side, and hyperresonance to percussion. Hypotension, marked tachycardia, cyanosis, and tracheal deviation raise suspicion for tension pneumothorax, which requires urgent interventions with needle decompression and possible chest tube placement [30, 34].

Diagnosis of pneumothorax can be made clinically, but confirmed with chest radiography. Lateral decubitus films with the affected side up are helpful in identifying small pneumothoraces in infants. Pneumothorax size is calculated by measuring the distance between the lung apex and the dome of thoracic cavity on the same side. A small pneumothorax is less than 3 cm, and large is greater than or equal to 3 cm [35]. Conservative management with observation (and sometimes supplemental oxygen) is recommended for clinically stable patients with small pneumothoraces, whereas clinically unstable patients and/or those with tension/large pneumothoraces require more aggressive intervention with needle decompression [34].

5.5 Prevention of RSV Infection

Palivizumab, a humanized monoclonal immunoglobulin antibody sold under the brand name of Synagis, is a prophylactic vaccine licensed by the Food and Drug Administration to reduce hospitalizations from serious lower respiratory tract infection caused by RSV in high-risk children [36]. Eligibility criteria for palivizumab are illustrated in Table 3. In qualifying infants and children, 5 monthly doses of palivizumab (15 mg/kg per dose) are recommended starting at the beginning of RSV season (November to April) [18, 36]. If an infant or child experiences breakthrough RSV hospitalization, monthly RSV prophylaxis is discontinued [36]. The baby described in this case would be eligible for palivizumab.

Table 3 Eligibility criteria for palivizumab prophylaxis

First year of life
Preterm infants born before **29 weeks gestation**
Preterm infants with **chronic lung disease (CLD) of prematurity** [1]
Infants with **acyanotic heart disease** receiving medication to control congestive heart failure and will require cardiac corrective surgery
Infants with **cardiac transplantation**
Infants with **moderate to severe pulmonary hypertension**
Second year of life
Infants with **CLD of prematurity**[a] requiring medical support[b] during 6 months before the start of the second RSV season
Infants with **cardiac transplantation**
May consider palivizumab prophylaxis, inadequate studies to definitively recommend prophylaxis
Infants with cyanotic heart disease[c]—first year of life
Infants with neuromuscular diseases or congenital anomalies that impair the ability of clear secretions—first year of life
Profoundly immunocompromised[d]—first and second years of life
Infants with cystic fibrosis with evidence of CLD and/or nutritional compromise—first year of life
Infants with cystic fibrosis with severe lung disease or weight for length <10th percentile—second year of life

[a] CLD of prematurity is defined as infants born at <32 weeks of gestation requiring >21% oxygen for at least the first 28 days after birth
[b] Chronic corticosteroid therapy, diuretic therapy, or supplemental oxygen
[c] Decision should be made in consultation with pediatric cardiologist
[d] As a result of chemotherapy, or hematopoietic, or solid-organ transplantation

6 Review Questions

1. An 8-week-old infant born at 36 weeks gestation presents to the hospital with 2 days of cough, congestion, low-grade fever, mildly increased work of breathing, and decreased wet diapers in a 24-h period. Vital signs include heart rate of 95 beats/min, respiratory rate of 63 breaths/min, blood pressure of 79/53 mmHg, and oxygen saturation of 91% on room air. Nasopharyngeal swab detects human rhinovirus.

   Of the following, the strongest indication for hospital admission for this patient is:

   (A) Fever in an 8-week-old patient
   (B) Respiratory effort
   (C) Oxygen saturation
   (D) Hydration status

2. A 6-month-old baby born at 27 weeks gestation with an extensive NICU course is seen in the emergency department for respiratory distress. Past medical history includes a 4-month NICU hospitalization that involved mechanical ventilation and CPAP, surfactant administration, caffeine for apnea, and phototherapy for jaundice, among others. The baby was discharged home on supplemental oxygen via nasal cannula and subsequently weaned to room air 3 weeks ago.

   Of the following, the postnatal intervention that most contributed to hindering this patient's respiratory function is:

   (A) Mechanical ventilation
   (B) Phototherapy
   (C) Surfactant administration
   (D) Continuous positive airway pressure ventilation

3. A 3-month-old baby with a history of persistent pulmonary hypertension of the newborn period presents to the emergency department in respiratory distress from viral bronchiolitis. As an emergency medicine provider, you suspect that the baby may be in pulmonary hypertensive crisis. Echocardiogram confirms right-to-left shunting.

   Of the following, which is NOT an appropriate treatment for an infant in pulmonary hypertensive crisis?

   (A) Supplemental 100% oxygen via nasal cannula
   (B) Inhaled nitric oxide at starting dose of 20 parts per million
   (C) Inhaled prostacyclin analog iloprost at starting dose of 2.5 μg
   (D) 0.9% sodium chloride bolus at 20 mL/kg over 15 min

4. A 7-month-old baby with a history of extreme prematurity at birth, bronchopulmonary dysplasia, and chronic lung disease presents to the emergency department in severe respiratory distress with oxygen saturations of 82% on room air. The baby does not improve with initial efforts of nasal cannula, high-flow nasal cannula, or continuous positive airway pressure. The baby is intubated for concern of impending respiratory arrest. Positive-pressure ventilation with bag-valve mask is provided prior to insertion of the endotracheal tube. Shortly after successful intubation evidenced by auscultation of breath sounds bilaterally, oxygen saturations drop again to 89%. Physical exam is notable for heart rate of 190 beats/min, blood pressure of 58/26 mmHg, and absent breath sounds of the left chest with hyperresonance to percussion.

   Of the following, the next best step is:

   (A) 100% FiO_2 oxygen
   (B) Anterior-posterior chest radiography
   (C) Needle decompression
   (D) Lateral decubitus chest radiography

7 Answers

1. **D**. Hydration status. Criteria for hospital admission for bronchiolitis include need for supplemental oxygen to maintain saturations >90%, decreased feeding volumes of ~50% of normal, dehydration, apnea, and significant respiratory distress. The infant's infection and congestion are likely hindering their ability to feed appropriately (in addition to increasing insensible fluid loss) as evidenced by the reported decreased number of wet diapers. Here, hydration status is the strongest indicator for this infant's hospital admission.
2. **A**. Mechanical ventilation. This is often necessary in order to adequately ventilate and oxygenate babies born prematurely. However, barotrauma and oxidative stress from invasive forms of ventilation can concurrently hinder normal development of lung parenchyma by facilitating fibrosis, smooth muscle hyperplasia, and abnormal alveolarization.
3. **D**. 0.9% Sodium chloride bolus at 20 mL/kg over 15 min. This would be inappropriate for an infant who presents with pulmonary hypertensive crisis as overly rapid fluid resuscitation may lead to fluid overload and worsening right-heart failure. Fluid administration should be in small aliquots of 5–10 mL/kg at a time with frequent reassessments before additional boluses are administered. 100% oxygen, inhaled nitric oxide, and prostacyclin analogs such as inhaled iloprost are all appropriate treatments for pulmonary hypertensive crisis that provide pulmonary vascular dilation and increased pulmonary blood flow.
4. **C**. Needle decompression. The baby is exhibiting signs of tension pneumothorax after receiving positive-pressure ventilation and mechanical ventilation. Tension pneumothorax is evidenced by signs of pneumothorax with hemodynamic instability. Chest radiographs may be done to support the diagnosis; however, given the patient's rapid development of hypotension and tachycardia, needle decompression is the next best step.

8 Takeaway Points

1. When evaluating a patient in respiratory distress, consider any significant past medical or birth history that can complicate the patient's clinical course.
2. Infants born prematurely with a history of bronchopulmonary dysplasia, chronic lung disease, congenital heart lesions, trisomy 21, and/or neuromuscular disease diagnosed with acute bronchiolitis are at high risk of apneic episodes and the need for aggressive respiratory support.
3. Bronchopulmonary dysplasia is one of the most common complications of preterm birth. Respiratory complications include increased airway resistance, reduced lung compliance, and air trapping, resulting in recurrent respiratory infections and exacerbations.

4. Pulmonary hypertensive crisis is a complication of acute illness in the setting of bronchopulmonary dysplasia and chronic lung disease. In addition to establishing adequate oxygenation, initial diagnostic evaluation includes electrocardiogram, chest radiograph, echocardiogram, and consultation with a pediatric cardiologist.
5. In pulmonary hypertensive crisis, goals of therapy encompass minimizing metabolic and hypoxic stress, optimizing ventilation, careful fluid resuscitation, supporting pulmonary vasodilation, and avoiding worsening right ventricular dysfunction.
6. Mechanical ventilation with high tidal volumes and high peak pressures increases the risk for barotrauma and pneumothorax.

References

1. Coalson JJ. Pathology of bronchopulmonary dysplasia. Semin Perinatol. 2006;30:179–84.
2. Jobe AH, Bancalari E. Bronchopulmonary dysplasia. Am J Respir Crit Care Med. 2001;163(7):1723–9.
3. Higgins R, et al. Bronchopulmonary dysplasia: executive summary of a workshop. J Pediatr. 2018;2018(197):300–8.
4. Abman SH, Mourani PM, Sontag M. Bronchopulmonary dysplasia: a genetic disease. Pediatrics. 2008;122(3).
5. Jobe AH. Mechanisms of lung injury and bronchopulmonary dysplasia. Am J Perinatol. 2016;33(11):1076–8.
6. Chess PR, D'Angio CT, Pryhuber GS, Maniscalco WM. Pathogenesis of bronchopulmonary dysplasia. Semin Perinatol. 2006;30(4):171–8. https://doi.org/10.1053/j.semperi.2006.05.003. PMID: 16860156
7. Yadav S, Lee B, Kamity R. Neonatal respiratory distress syndrome. Treasure Island: StatPearls Publishing; 2023.
8. Jobe AH. The new BPD: an arrest of lung development. Pediatr Res. 1999;46:641.
9. Jobe AH, Steinhorn R. Can we define bronchopulmonary dysplasia? J Pediatr. 2017;2017:19–23.
10. Alvarez-Fuente M, et al. Preventing bronchopulmonary dysplasia: new tools for an old challenge. Pediatr Res. 2018;85(4):432–41.
11. Manley BJ, Owen LS, Doyle LW, Andersen CC, Cartwright DW, Pritchard MA, Donath SM, Davis PG. High-flow nasal cannulae in very preterm infants after extubation. N Engl J Med. 2013;369(15):1425–33.
12. Askie LM, Darlow BA, Davis PG, Finer N, Stenson B, Vento M, Whyte R. Effects of targeting lower versus higher arterial oxygen saturations on death or disability in preterm infants. Cochrane Database Syst Rev. 2017;4(4):CD011190.
13. Davidson LM, Berkelhamer SK. Bronchopulmonary dysplasia: chronic lung disease of infancy and long-term pulmonary outcomes. J Clin Med. 2017;6(1):4.
14. Jobe AH. The new bronchopulmonary dysplasia. Curr Opin Pediatr. 2011;23(2):167–72.
15. Katz TA, et al. Severity of bronchopulmonary dysplasia and neurodevelopmental outcome at 2 and 5 years corrected age. J Pediatr. 2022;2018(243):40–46.e2.
16. Karampatsas K, Kong J, Cohen J. Bronchiolitis: an update on management and prophylaxis. Br J Hosp Med. 2019;80(5):278–84.
17. Florin TA, Plint AC, Zore JJ. Viral bronchiolitis. Lancet. 2017;389(10065):211–24. https://doi.org/10.1016/S0140-6736(16)30951-5.
18. Ralston SL, Lieberthal AS, Meissner HC, et al. Clinical practice guideline: the diagnosis, management, and prevention of bronchiolitis. Pediatrics. 2014;134(5):e1474–502.
19. Barron Frazier S, Walls C, Jain S, Plemmons G, Johnson DP. Reducing chest radiographs in bronchiolitis through high-reliability interventions. Pediatrics. 2021;148(3):e2020014597. https://doi.org/10.1542/peds.2020-014597.

20. Walsh-Sukys MC, Tyson JE, Wright LL, Bauer CR, Korones SB, Stevenson DK, et al. Persistent pulmonary hypertension of the newborn in the era before nitric oxide: practice variation and outcomes. Pediatrics. 2000;105:14–20.
21. Hernandez-Diaz S, Van Marter LJ, Werler MM, Louik C, Mitchell AA. Risk factors for persistent pulmonary hypertension. Pediatrics. 2007;120:e272–82.
22. Lakshminrusimha S, Steinhorn RH. Pulmonary vascular biology during neonatal transition. Clin Perinatol. 1999;26(3):601–19.
23. Teitel DF, Iwamoto HS, Rudolph AM. Changes in the pulmonary circulation during birth-related events. Pediatr Res. 1990;27:372–8.
24. Crossley KJ, Allison BJ, Polglase GR, Morley CJ, Davis PG, Hooper SB. Dynamic changes in the direction of blood flow through the ductus arteriosus at birth. J Physiol. 2009;587:4695–704.
25. Rosenzweig EB, Abman SH, Adatia I, Beghetti M, Bonnet D, Haworth S, et al. Paediatric pulmonary arterial hypertension: updates on definition, classification, diagnostics and management. Eur Respir J. 2019;53:1801916.
26. Rosenzweig EB, Feinstein JA, Humpl T, et al. Pulmonary arterial hypertension in children: diagnostic work-up and challenges. Prog Pediatr Cardiol. 2009;27:7–11.
27. Bendapudi P, Rao GG, Greenough A. Diagnosis and management of persistent pulmonary hypertension of the newborn. Paediatr Respir Rev. 2015;16(3):157–61.
28. Benedict N, Seybert A, Mathier MA. Evidence-based pharmacologic management of pulmonary arterial hypertension. Clin Ther. 2007;29:2134–53.
29. Abman SH, Hansmann G, Archer SL, et al. Pediatric pulmonary hypertension: guidelines from the American Heart Association and American Thoracic Society [published correction appears in Circulation. 2016 Jan 26;133(4):e368]. Circulation. 2015;132(21):2037–99.
30. Posner K, Needleman JP. Pneumothorax. Pediatr Rev. 2008;29(2):69–70. https://doi.org/10.1542/pir.29-2-69.
31. Gomella TL, et al. Pneumothorax. In: Neonatology: management, procedures, on-call problems, diseases, and drugs. 7th ed. New York: McGraw Hill; 2013.
32. Silva D, Sérgio P, et al. Iatrogenic pneumothorax in mechanically ventilated children: incidence, risk factors and other outcomes. Heart Lung. 2015;44(3):238–42. https://doi.org/10.1016/j.hrtlng.2015.01.005.
33. Miller JD, Carlo WA. Pulmonary complications of mechanical ventilation in neonates. Clin Perinatol. 2008;35(1):273–81. https://doi.org/10.1016/j.clp.2007.11.004.
34. Goldman RD. Spontaneous pneumothorax in children. Can Fam Physician. 2020;66(10):737–8.
35. Baumann MH, et al. Management of spontaneous pneumothorax. Chest. 2001;119(2):590–602. https://doi.org/10.1378/chest.119.2.590.
36. Brady MT, et al. Updated guidance for palivizumab prophylaxis among infants and young children at increased risk of hospitalization for respiratory syncytial virus infection. Pediatrics. 2014;134(2):415–20. https://doi.org/10.1542/peds.2014-1665.

Further Readings

Davidson LM, Berkelhamer SK. Bronchopulmonary dysplasia: chronic lung disease of infancy and long-term pulmonary outcomes. J Clin Med. 2017;6(1):4.

Rosenzweig EB, Abman SH, Adatia I, Beghetti M, Bonnet D, Haworth S, et al. Paediatric pulmonary arterial hypertension: updates on definition, classification, diagnostics and management. Eur Respir J. 2019;53:1801916.

Silva D, Sérgio P, et al. Iatrogenic pneumothorax in mechanically ventilated children: incidence, risk factors and other outcomes. Heart Lung. 2015;44(3):238–42. https://doi.org/10.1016/j.hrtlng.2015.01.005.

Silver AH, Nazif JM. Bronchiolitis. Pediatr Rev. 2019;40(11):568–76.

Fever in a Patient with Short Bowel Syndrome

Rebecca Tenney-Soeiro and Christina Bales

1 Case

A 17-month-old male with GERD and parenteral nutrition (PN)-dependent short bowel syndrome presents to the emergency department with lethargy and fever after several days of intermittent abdominal distention, diarrhea, and vomiting.

He was born at 33 weeks to a healthy G1P0 mother whose prenatal ultrasound demonstrated polyhydramnios with dilated fetal bowel. Abdominal exploration on day 2 of life revealed a type IIIB jejunal atresia with small bowel volvulus and ischemia. After several abdominal surgeries, he was left with only 25 cm of jejunum anastomosed to his transverse colon. Diarrhea limited enteral feeding, and so he was discharged to home on a combination of gastrostomy feeds and PN delivered via a tunneled central venous catheter.

He was in his usual state of health until 6 days ago, when he developed increased abdominal distention and foul flatulence, followed by bouts of watery diarrhea and bile-tinged emesis. This morning, he was unusually sleepy and had an isolated temperature to 38.6 °C, prompting presentation. He has no cough, congestion, or sick contacts. Medications include omeprazole, cholestyramine, and enoxaparin.

On examination: temperature 37.2 °C, pulse 137, BP 105/65, RR 22, and O_2 Sat 98% on RA. He arouses with vigorous stimulation. He has tacky mucous membranes with mild tachycardia. Lungs are clear. The central line insertion site is clean and dry and covered with a sterile dressing. The abdomen has well-healed scars and a G-tube with no surrounding skin changes. His abdomen is moderately distended, tympanic, compressible, and non-tender. A firm liver extends 4 cm below the costal margin. The spleen is not palpable.

R. Tenney-Soeiro (✉) · C. Bales
Department of Pediatrics, Children's Hospital of Philadelphia, Philadelphia, PA, USA
e-mail: tenneysoeiro@chop.edu; balesc@chop.edu

A. Kamzan et al. (eds.), *Children with Medical Complexity in the Emergency Department*, https://doi.org/10.1007/978-3-031-62517-6_11

Testing:

CBC: WBC 11.1/Hb 12.2/Hgb 12.0/Plt 266
CMP: Na 137/K 4.0/Cl 107/HCO3 13/BUN 10/Creat 0.2/glucose 58/T Bili 1.2/albumin 4.4/ALT 125/AST 130/GGT 200
UA: SG 1.030; otherwise negative
Abdominal X-ray: Multiple air-fluid levels. No distention of small bowel to suggest high-grade obstruction

2 Discussion Questions

1. What parts of the history and physical exam guide your clinical decision-making and differential diagnosis in this patient?
2. What are common and uncommon complications of short bowel syndrome throughout childhood?

3 Case Answers

1. His short bowel syndrome (SBS) and need for PN with a central line, documented fever at home, and diarrhea with potentially bilious emesis are key components of his history. His physical exam findings of sleepiness, tachycardia, hepatomegaly, and abdominal distention with air fluid levels on X-ray are concerning. Notable laboratory findings include acidosis, hypoglycemia, and modest elevations in liver enzymes including GGT. The differential diagnosis should include infection (including *c*entral *l*ine-*a*ssociated *b*loodstream *i*nfection = CLABSI), dehydration with hypoglycemia (some component of this due to vomiting/diarrhea), partial bowel obstruction, *s*mall *i*ntestinal *b*acterial *o*vergrowth syndrome (SIBO) with possible concomitant D-lactic acidosis, medication or other toxin exposure (e.g., cholestyramine can cause acidosis), pancreatitis, and choledocholithiasis, cholecystitis, or other biliary complication.
2. Complications of SBS may be related to the underlying abnormal gastrointestinal (GI) tract and nutritional vulnerability, to parenteral nutrition and/or other medications, and to central lines (if present). Patients are at increased risk for feeding intolerance, which may manifest with vomiting, diarrhea, and/or bloating and may be associated with dehydration or hypoglycemia. These symptoms may be disproportionately exacerbated by infection, SIBO, or complications of previous surgeries (adhesions, strictures). Patients are at risk for a broad range of vitamin and mineral deficiencies and associated complications. While parenteral nutrition may decrease these risks, it introduces other substantial risks, including liver disease, biliary and pancreatic complications, and collateral challenges

associated with the central venous catheter needed for PN administration. Indeed, the combination of the central line and PN involves extreme vulnerability to line-associated infections. Patients are also vulnerable to central venous thrombosis and loss of venous access over time. In this case, the treating provider should think about infection, especially CLABSI, and the rare, but cannot miss, diagnosis of small intestinal bacterial overgrowth syndrome with D-lactic acidosis.

4 Learning Objectives

1. Explain the pathophysiology of short bowel syndrome.
2. Describe the complications of short bowel syndrome.
3. Understand the initial management of fever and increased stool output in short bowel syndrome.
4. Recognize D-lactic acidosis due to small intestinal bacterial overgrowth.

5 Discussion

Children with short bowel syndrome (SBS) have insufficient functional bowel to absorb the nutrients and fluid needed for adequate growth, hydration, and electrolyte balance. Most pediatric cases of SBS evolve in the perinatal period. Premature babies are predominantly affected, and recent improvements in perinatal care have led to improved survival of premature infants that has translated into a rapidly expanding pediatric short bowel population.

Affected infants may have congenital short bowel length (e.g., intestinal atresia, gastroschisis) or compromised bowel function (e.g., long-segment Hirschsprung disease). Alternatively, they may suffer devastating loss of the intestines due to necrotizing enterocolitis or less common entities, such as meconium ileus or volvulus. Later in childhood, bowel loss is unusual, but can occur due to rare events, including trauma, neoplasm, sepsis, or particularly aggressive Crohn disease. Regardless of the etiology, SBS tends to occur in the context of medical complexity, and children with SBS therefore require a detailed and thoughtful approach to differential diagnosis and management when presenting to the emergency department.

Patients with SBS often rely upon intravenous or "parenteral" nutrition (PN) to survive and thrive. PN is a mixture of water, electrolytes, dextrose, and amino acids, which may also be supplemented with lipid emulsion, vitamins, and minerals. It is typically delivered through a sterile tunneled catheter that enters the chest wall, cannulates a central vein, and terminates near the right atrium of the heart. Central administration of PN is critical due to its high osmolality, which may damage peripheral veins. Even with appropriate central administration of PN, children with SBS remain at high risk for venous thrombosis and loss of vascular access points.

Over time, children with SBS may be able to slowly transition from parenteral to enteral and/or oral nutrition. In the youngest patients, this transition may be facilitated by physiologic intestinal lengthening with maturity. Indeed, the normal human small bowel doubles in length during the last trimester of pregnancy, and it then triples in length in the first 5 years of life [1]. Most young children with SBS retain some of this growth capacity. Patients with SBS may also experience “intestinal adaptation,” a compensatory phenomenon in which small bowel mucosal mass increases and permits more efficient absorption. This adaptive process may be facilitated by enteral feeding, endogenous hormones, and certain medications (e.g., teduglutide). In select cases, surgeries can be performed to reconstruct the bowel to promote more efficient nutrient and fluid absorption. These surgeries, such as the serial transverse enteroplasty procedure (STEP), essentially exchange bowel width for bowel length and aim to augment mucosal surface area for absorption and improve bowel function. Ultimately, the goal of intestinal rehabilitation is enteral autonomy. Factors which predict independence from PN include longer small intestine length, greater degree of prematurity, a diagnosis of NEC, and retention of the ileocecal valve [2]. In rare cases, in which enteral autonomy cannot be achieved and children experience untenable complications of PN, such as loss of central venous access and advanced liver disease, intestinal transplantation may be considered.

Children with SBS experience a variety of gastrointestinal symptoms at baseline, and these symptoms must be distinguished from acute symptoms. Chronic diarrhea is common and multifactorial. Short bowel length is inherently associated with a reduced intestinal mucosal surface area for fluid absorption, which causes diarrhea. Fecal loss may also be compounded by physiologic changes that are driven by the specific distribution of missing bowel. For example, patients with jejunostomies or ileostomies may be vulnerable to rapid intestinal transit due to loss of endogenous hormones produced by cells in the terminal ileum that regulate peristalsis. In patients with terminal ileal resection and small bowel-colon anastomosis, enterohepatic recirculation of bile acids may be disrupted, leading to excessive delivery of bile acids to the colon, where bacteria cause bile acid deconjugation that, in turn, promotes a “bile acid” diarrhea.

In addition to diarrhea, patients with SBS may suffer from abdominal bloating and vomiting. Previous abdominal surgeries with sometimes multiple bowel anastomoses can predispose to adhesions, strictures, or regions of altered bowel motility that can potentiate bowel dilation and emesis. Distinguishing chronic anatomic differences from acute changes that may herald frank intestinal obstruction or other surgical emergencies can be especially challenging. A careful history, which focuses on differentiating new or recently escalated signs and symptoms from baseline features, is critical. Referencing any previous imaging that may be available can also be helpful.

Like all children, pediatric SBS patients experience common illnesses, but they often experience more exaggerated gastrointestinal sequelae than their healthy counterparts. Even ubiquitous viral infections may be associated with exuberant and protracted gastrointestinal losses. Diarrhea may predispose to urinary tract infection, especially in female and diapered patients, and the presence of a central line introduces a risk of serious infections. Infections can include a superficial cellulitis at the insertion site, a tunnel infection which extends into the soft tissues surrounding the catheter (typically detected with ultrasound in the setting of skin erythema, swelling, or purulence), and bacteremia. Indeed, children with PN-dependent SBS represent one of the highest risk groups for *c*entral line-*a*ssociated *b*loodstream *i*nfections (CLABSIs), which may present with fever, lethargy, altered consciousness, tachycardia, or other cardiovascular instability. Early presentations of CLABSI may be subtle, and even subjective parental report of fever at home should trigger a high suspicion for CLABSI in this population.

While lifesaving for patients with SBS, PN can also be associated with complications. Intestinal failure-associated liver disease (IFALD) is common and can manifest with cholestasis, hepatitis, or some combination thereof. A lack of enteral feeding, sometimes coupled with the aforementioned disruption of bile acid circulation, can also potentiate biliary stasis, which can compound hepatic injury and lead to cholecystitis, cholelithiasis, choledocholithiasis, and even gallstone pancreatitis. With prolonged PN exposure, liver disease may advance to involve portal hypertension with attendant risk for bleeding from gastric or esophageal varices. Bleeding may also be potentiated by coagulopathy due to liver synthetic dysfunction or deficiencies in vitamins, including vitamin K. Other important sources of gastrointestinal bleeding in this population include anastomotic ulcers and side effects of medications. Anticoagulants, used to prevent central line-associated deep vein thrombosis, are common culprits.

Small intestinal bacterial overgrowth (SIBO) syndrome is another important complication of SBS. The shorter small intestine length, often with lack of the ileocecal valve, augments the delivery of undigested nutrients to colonic bacteria and fuels their proliferation. Intestinal stasis in dilated bowel loops and proton pump inhibitor use may also increase the risk for this phenomenon. Hydrogen and/or methane gas produced by bacteria may lead to abdominal distention and foul flatulence with or without vomiting. Recent evidence suggests that patients with SBS—and particularly those on PN—have decreased intestinal bacterial diversity and are more likely to harbor pro-inflammatory bacteria that can cause mucosal injury, which can exacerbate diarrhea and malabsorption [3]. Bacterial overgrowth may also theoretically predispose to translocation of bacteria to the bloodstream.

In select cases, patients with SBS and SIBO may be colonized with D-lactic acid-forming organisms. When such patients consume large quantities of carbohydrates, these organisms can ferment undigested carbohydrates in the colon to D-lactic acid, which can cause a profound acidosis that may be accompanied by lethargy and altered mental status, ataxia, and dysarthria. In young, nonverbal, and non-ambulating children, neurologic symptoms may be subtle, and lethargy may be the only appreciable clue to this elusive entity. D-lactate, which is almost uniquely produced by bacteria, requires a special assay, and it is not identified with standard lactate assays, which are designed to identify L-lactate, the primary human isomer of lactate. Thus, clinicians must have a heightened awareness of this entity in children with SBS and have a low threshold to suspect it as a potential culprit for metabolic acidosis in this population. Special blood D-lactate levels, if available to the clinician, should be submitted. However, treatment typically needs to be initiated before these levels result [4, 5].

6 Differential Diagnosis

In this case of a premature toddler with SBS presenting with fever and lethargy after nearly a week of abdominal bloating, foul flatulence, intermittent vomiting, and diarrhea, the differential should include a broad range of infections: viral, urinary tract, and—most importantly—CLABSI. Small intestinal bacterial overgrowth, which commonly involves the prodromal features that evolved in the days preceding his presentation, is an important consideration. Biliary complications should also be included in the differential, particularly in light of abnormal liver transaminases (which could also be his baseline labs). Hypoglycemia and dehydration due to excessive GI losses may compound the presentation. Finally, medication toxicity (e.g., cholestyramine) and vitamin deficiency (e.g., thiamine deficiency) must be considered, particularly as potential culprits of metabolic acidosis.

7 Management

Initial steps in the management of this lethargic child should include a finger-stick blood glucose and correction of the low level with dextrose, followed by collection of laboratory studies and fluid resuscitation beginning with 20 mL/kg of normal saline (NS) or lactated Ringer's (LR). In addition to the basic studies presented in the case, labs should include a blood culture from the central line, stool infectious studies, toxicology screen, fractionated bilirubin level, amylase, lipase, a thiamine level, and—if possible—a D-lactate level. Tachycardia and acidosis with reported GI losses should prompt NPO status until cardiovascular stability and electrolyte balance are achieved. Children with SBS often require greater than maintenance fluids at baseline, and the patient's home regimen (PN + EN) should be taken into account when developing a fluid plan. If vomiting persists, the G-tube should be drained to gravity with careful accounting of losses, and a sump should be placed if this does not alleviate symptoms. The global presentation in the context of a reported temperature >38 °C at home warrants prompt initiation of broad-spectrum antibiotics to cover both gram-positive and gram-negative culprits of bacteremia (e.g., a third-generation cephalosporin and vancomycin) for at least 48 h pending culture results. IV thiamine administration is also prudent. Finally, the elevated bilirubin level and liver transaminases should prompt consideration of an ultrasound of the abdomen, particularly if some of the aforementioned labs raise suspicion for biliary or pancreatic complications. Serial abdominal exams should be performed, and higher level imaging and surgical input considered if tenderness or other concerning features evolve.

8 Case Outcome

Fluid resuscitation with NPO status resulted in rapid resolution (<24 h) of symptoms and restoration of electrolyte balance. Pancreatic enzyme levels were normal, an ultrasound was reassuring outside of baseline hepatomegaly, and blood cultures revealed no growth of organisms. In collaboration with the patient's primary GI doctor, the home feeding regimen was adjusted to minimize simple carbohydrates and avoid continuous feeds, which could fuel overgrowth of bacteria. An enteral antibiotic targeting common D-lactate-producing bacteria (e.g., enteral metronidazole) was initiated. With these changes, the patient's baseline status was restored. One week later, the D-lactate level confirmed the diagnosis of D-lactic acidosis (D-lactate 1.9; normal 0–0.26) in the setting of clinical features of SIBO.

9 Review Questions

1. What is a necessary step in a patient with short bowel syndrome and PN dependence who presents to the emergency department with a fever?
   (A) Obtain an abdominal X-ray
   (B) Obtain a blood culture from the central line and start broad-spectrum antibiotics
   (C) Discontinue all enteral feeds
   (D) Obtain a urine culture
2. D-lactic acid production is increased in short bowel patients due to what mechanism?
   (A) Fast transit time in the intestine leads to decreased fat absorption
   (B) Carbohydrate malabsorption leads to an overgrowth of bacteria
   (C) Vitamin deficiencies prevent the normal breakdown of D-lactic acid in the colon
   (D) The cholestasis associated with PN leads to an increase in D-lactic acid in the blood
3. Which of the following is not associated with small intestine bacterial overgrowth (SIBO)?
   (A) Loose stools
   (B) Malabsorption
   (C) Rash
   (D) Abdominal distention

10 Answers

1. **B.** A child who has a central line and presents with temperature ≥38.0 °C should always have a blood culture obtained from the central line and given broad-spectrum antibiotics. Typical regimens broadly cover both gram-positive and gram-negative culprits (e.g., third-generation cephalosporin and vancomycin). Antifungal coverage may be added in cases of cardiovascular instability, particularly if vasopressors are needed. An abdominal X-ray and urine culture may be obtained in some situations but are not necessary in every patient. If the child is tolerating enteral feeds, there is no need to discontinue the enteral feeds in the setting of fever.
2. **B.** Shortened small intestine can lead to malabsorption of carbohydrates, fats, and vitamins. It is the carbohydrate malabsorption which promotes the growth of bacteria that may contain D-lactate dehydrogenase, thus leading to an increase in D-lactic acid production. While PN usage is associated with a shorter small intestine, its use does not directly lead to the presence of D-lactic acid in the blood.
3. **C**. SIBO is often associated with abdominal distention, foul-smelling flatulence, loose stools, and occasionally emesis. A rash is not associated with SIBO and in the setting of loose stools may be more suggestive of a food protein allergy.

11 Takeaway Points

1. The pediatric SBS population is growing as the neonatal population grows due to improved perinatal care, and familiarity with SBS is important for pediatric ED physicians and hospitalists.
2. Pediatric SBS typically occurs in the context of medical complexity and warrants careful consideration of multiple contributing factors.
3. Typical symptoms of common childhood illness, such as fever, vomiting, and diarrhea, have a broad differential in the SBS patient that necessitates familiarity with the underlying pathophysiology of SBS and a thoughtful interpretation of subtle features.
4. The risk of CLABSI in the PN-dependent SBS population exceeds that of other line-dependent populations and mandates a high index of suspicion for this entity.
5. D-lactic acidosis is a rare finding in patients with SBS due to challenges in measuring D-lactate in most clinical settings, and it requires a high index of clinical suspicion to render a timely diagnosis.

References

1. Strugis MC, Diamond IR, deSilva N. Establishing norms for intestinal length in children. J Pediatr Surg. 2009;44:933–8.
2. Khan FA, Squires RH, Litman HJ, et al. Predictors of enteral autonomy in children with intestinal failure: a multicenter cohort study. J Pediatr. 2015;167:29–34.
3. Piper HG, Coughlin LA, Nguyen V, et al. A comparison of small bowel and fecal microbiota in children with short bowel syndrome. J Pediatr Surg. 2020;55:878–82.
4. Petersen C. D-lactic acidosis. Nutr Clin Pract. 2005;20:634–45.
5. Goulet O, Nader EA, Pigneur B, Lambe C. Short bowel syndrome as the leading cause of intestinal failure in early life: some insights into the management. Pediatr Gastroeneterol Hepatol Nutri. 2019;22(4):303–29. https://doi.org/10.5223/pghn.2019.22.4.303.

A Child with Bleeding from a Tracheostomy Tube

James A. Lin and Alisha N. West

1 Case

A 6-year-old girl is brought to the emergency department (ED) for evaluation of bloody tracheal secretions. Her history is notable for nonfatal drowning at the age of 2, leading to chronic hypoxic ischemic encephalopathy, global developmental delay, and generalized spasticity. She is dependent on mechanical ventilation via tracheostomy tube and enteral feeds via gastrostomy tube. Her caretakers note that she frequently hyperextends her neck, a behavior that has been presumed to be a sign of gastroesophageal reflux. Yesterday, the patient developed an episode of bright red blood suctioned from her tracheostomy tube, which resolved with conservative care using cold saline instillation and red rubber suction catheters. This afternoon, another episode of bright red blood was noted upon routine tracheostomy tube suctioning. Bleeding persisted despite conservative measures. In the ED, the patient is tachycardic and afebrile with otherwise normal vital signs. Her ventilator support is at baseline. Upon initial respiratory therapist assessment, the tracheostomy tube cuff is found to be inflated to a pressure of 40 cmH_2O and is adjusted down to 20 cmH_2O. Chest X-ray reveals the tip of the tracheostomy tube in the mid-trachea and nonspecific findings suggestive of multifocal atelectasis versus airspace disease. Empiric antibiotics are initiated. During physician assessment, the tracheostomy tube is seen to beat subtly in time with the heart rate. Shortly, bright red, pulsatile blood is ejected from the stoma, and the patient desaturates as the ventilator alarms.

J. A. Lin (✉)
Department of Pediatrics, University of California Los Angeles, Los Angeles, CA, USA
e-mail: jameslin@mednet.ucla.edu

A. N. West
Department of Head and Neck Surgery, University of California Los Angeles,
Los Angeles, CA, USA
e-mail: awest@mednet.ucla.edu

A. Kamzan et al. (eds.), *Children with Medical Complexity in the Emergency Department*, https://doi.org/10.1007/978-3-031-62517-6_12

While awaiting operating room availability for emergent otolaryngology and thoracic surgery intervention, the doctor considers how to contain the bleeding.

2 Discussion Questions

1. What causes of tracheal bleeding must be considered at initial presentation in this case?
2. What interventions might temporize rapid bleeding in this case, pending definitive surgical intervention?

3 Case Answers

1. Sources of bleeding from an established tracheostomy include tracheal granulation tissue, suction trauma of tracheal epithelium, tracheo-vascular fistula, inflamed tracheal epithelium from tracheitis, bronchial arteries in the lower respiratory tree, and pulmonary alveolar hemorrhage. Tracheoinnominate artery fistula can present as a "sentinel bleed": self-limited, bright red bleeding preceding a major hemorrhage. Pulsation of the tracheostomy or tube is another early sign.
2. Direct pressure on a tracheoinnominate artery fistula can be applied by (i) displacing the tube to position the cuff over the area of hemorrhage and hyperinflating the cuff or (ii) through direct digital pressure using the Utley maneuver.

4 Learning Objectives

1. Understand the risk factors for tracheal bleeding in patients with tracheostomy tubes.
2. Describe the fundamental tracheostomy tube management decisions that affect the risk of tracheal bleeding.
3. Understand the initial management of hemorrhage from a tracheoinnominate artery fistula.

5 Discussion

5.1 Definitions and Epidemiology

In this chapter, we will use the term *tracheotomy* to refer to the surgical procedure that allows insertion of a breathing tube via an opening in the trachea and *tracheostomy* for the resultant opening traversing the skin into the trachea [1]. The

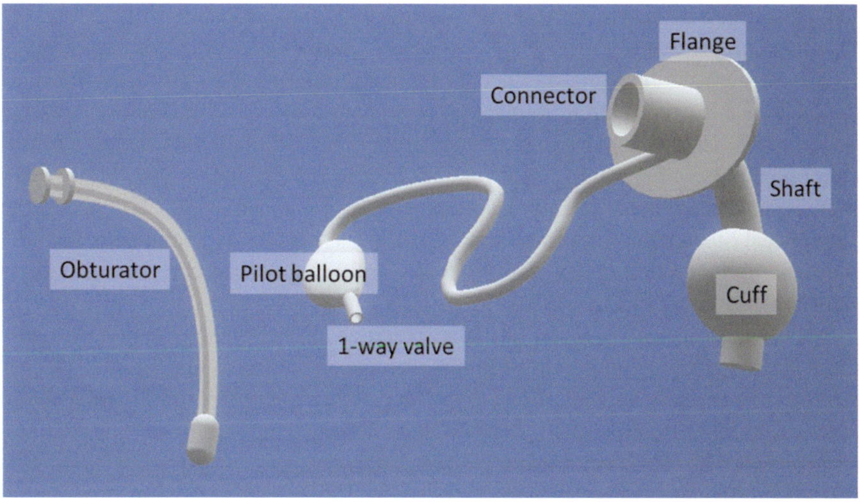

Fig. 1 Components of a tracheostomy tube

components of a standard tracheostomy tube are shown in Fig. 1. We will describe complications of these tubes that lead to bleeding.

Tracheostomy tubes are frequently seen in hospitalized children. More than 4800 tracheotomies are performed annually in pediatric patients [2], the majority of whom have multiple medical comorbidities [3, 4]. Almost 2% of pediatric intensive care unit patients receive a tracheostomy tube [5]. In 2009, there were 21,541 hospitalizations for children with preexisting tracheostomy tubes, the majority of whom were discharged home [4]. Tracheostomy complications are commonly reported in these hospitalizations, including tracheostomy hemorrhage (3.4%), infection of tracheostomy (1.6%), and tracheal stenosis (1.1%) [4].

5.2 *Blood in Tracheal Secretions*

The presence of blood in tracheal secretions is a common complaint among children with long-term tracheostomy tubes. In the early postoperative period, defined as 7 days or less postoperatively, bleeding is one of the most common adverse events after pediatric tracheotomy, occurring in approximately 0–5.2% [6–10]. Capillary ooze due to inadequate surgical hemostasis is usually the cause in the early postoperative period and may necessitate surgical revision [3, 10]. While coagulopathy is a theoretical risk factor for post-tracheotomy bleeding [11], associated conditions like hepatic failure and thrombocytopenia are usually known or suspected preoperatively and addressed [2, 3]. In the first 2 years after tracheostomy for children on Medicaid, 39% experienced a tracheostomy-related complication, more than a third of which were due to hemorrhage or tracheoesophageal fistula [12]. A case series of 1094 surveillance direct laryngoscopy and bronchoscopy (DLB) in children with tracheostomies noted pre-procedural bleeding in 2% of procedures [13]. Tracheal bleeding can present as blood-tinged secretions, hemoptysis, or major hemorrhage. Late postoperative bleeding, defined as bleeding more than 7 days after tracheotomy, can result from suction trauma [14], stomal granuloma or tracheal granulation tissue [6, 12, 15–17], and tracheoarterial fistula [14]. Although inflammation of tracheobronchial epithelium by infection can lead to minor bleeding [3, 11, 18, 19], blood-tinged secretions are not a common sign of tracheitis [20, 21]. Along the same lines, bleeding from a tracheostomy tube can present as hemoptysis due to a pulmonary, lower respiratory tree, or even esophageal source, but these presentations are unusual [18, 22].

Granulation tissue is one of the most common late complications of tracheostomy tubes requiring intervention [9] and a common source of bleeding [23], especially when injured by suctioning. Formed in response to friction, foreign body reaction, suction trauma, and infection, granulation tissue is initially soft, friable, and vascular [23, 24]. Histologically, granulation tissue is composed of blood vessels, macrophages, and inflammatory cells [25]. Superficial ulceration is common. As granulation tissue epithelializes and is replaced by fibrous tissue, it is termed an intraluminal granuloma [26]. The suprastomal location at the cephalad aspect of the internal stoma site is the most common area for granuloma growth [24]. Granulation tissue is frequently observed at tracheotomy, having developed secondary to prior translaryngeal (oral) endotracheal intubation [6, 26]. Granuloma formation may occur as soon as a week after tracheotomy but usually requires weeks to years to develop. In recent case series of children with tracheostomy tubes undergoing DLB, granulomas or granulation tissue are observed in 38–44% [13, 16], though earlier reports noted them in as many as 50–100% of pediatric patients [6, 26]. Tracheal granulation tissue has been observed to grow through the fenestrations of a tracheostomy tube, causing obstruction and inability to decannulate [15, 27]. In a series of 1094 DLBs in pediatric patients with tracheostomy tube, debridement of a suprastomal granuloma was the most common intervention and performed in 41% [13]. The mean time to first excision of granuloma after tracheotomy is approximately 14 months [24]. Because tracheal granulomas are so common and recur frequently after surgical excision [26], judgment must be exercised about when to intervene [3]. Both granulation tissue and granulomas are associated with tracheal bleeding. Treatment of tracheal granulation can include topical antibiotics and/or steroids, chemical (silver nitrate) or electrical cautery, or sharp or laser excision [3, 16, 17]. Custom-length tracheostomy tubes may be required to bypass tracheal granulation [16, 17]. Because granulation tissue forms in response to epithelial contact with the tube, downsizing the tracheostomy tube might also help [26].

Suction trauma is well-recognized as a cause of bloody tracheal aspirates [3, 14, 18]. The technique of suctioning tracheostomy tubes is critical to maintain a clear airway while avoiding undue airway injury. One common practice is to limit suctioning to within the tracheostomy tube and no further than the tip, but national consensus statements differ. An American Thoracic Society (ATS) statement recommends routine use of the "premeasured technique," in which suction tubing with side holes near the distal tip is inserted only deep enough into the tracheostomy tube for the distal holes to just exit the tip of the tube [14]. This strategy is meant to avoid denuding tracheal epithelium and causing inflammation that can exacerbate airway injury and elicit bleeding or formation of granulation tissue. Conversely, accurate depth of suctioning ensures that the tracheostomy tube is adequately cleared of obstructing mucus. A more recent American Academy of Otolaryngology-Head and Neck Surgery (AAO-HNS) consensus panel was unable to reach consensus to prescribe the depth of tracheal tube suctioning, citing lack of definitive data [1]. Further recommendations by the ATS to optimize tracheal tube suctioning include the following: (i) use of the largest caliber tube that will fit through the tracheostomy tube to facilitate efficient clearance, (ii) limiting the amount of time spent in active suctioning to less than 5 s, and (iii) twirling or rotating the suction catheter between fingers and thumb, not stirring the catheter with the entire hand. These measures balance the goal of clearing the airway adequately versus the possible untoward effects of negative-pressure injury to the epithelium and atelectasis caused by occlusion of the tracheostomy tube and the negative pressure of suctioning. Use of soft red rubber suction catheters to reduce catheter-related trauma is a common recommendation [18].

Warming and humidifying inspired gases via the tracheostomy tube is a standard practice, meant to prevent tube plugging by dried or clotted secretions and facilitate airway clearance by suctioning or spontaneous coughing [28]. For patients using heat-and-moisture exchange ("HME") devices for humidification, some recommend transitioning to a mist collar mask for humidification when mucus is blood-tinged [3]. Unfortunately, evidence in favor of either active or passive humidification to prevent device-related complications is lacking [28]. Based on physiologic data on the normal temperature and humidity of air in the upper airway, the ATS recommends that inspired gas be warmed to a temperature of 32–34 °C and humidified to 36–40 mg/L.

5.3 *Decision to Use Tracheostomy Tube Cuff*

Tracheostomy tube cuffs are inflatable balloons surrounding the tube tip that are used to occlude the space between the tube and the tracheal wall. Use of an inflated cuff allows efficient transmission of airway pressure and inspired gas volume by limiting leakage around the tube [28]. Tracheostomy tube cuffs are commonly used to facilitate mechanical ventilation and airway clearance in adult and pediatric patients. Differences in manufacture and design of tracheostomy tube cuff preclude all but a few simple recommendations on their use. Cuffs can be characterized by low-pressure or high-pressure, air-filled or water-filled, low-volume or high-volume, or foam design [28]. Indications for use of a tracheostomy tube cuff are thought to be patient specific, and evidence supporting one practice over another for when to use a cuff is lacking [1]. One theoretical benefit of a tracheostomy tube cuff is to reduce aspiration of irritant liquids like gastroesophageal or laryngopharyngeal reflux into the lungs, but pooling of those same liquids above an inflated cuff can cause chemical injury and exacerbate previous airway damage [23]. Furthermore, the benefit of the cuff to reducing clinically significant aspiration is limited. Multiple carefully designed imaging studies demonstrated that 30–50% of mechanically ventilated patients with an inflated or deflated tracheostomy tube cuff experience intermittent aspiration [23, 29–31].

Tracheal stenosis most commonly develops at the tracheostoma but is also described at the site of a cuff or tube tip [23]. Low-volume high-pressure tube cuffs have largely been replaced by high-volume low-pressure designs over the years, with benefits in reducing the risk for tracheal stenosis [23]. Still, overinflation or excessive pressure of the tube cuff above capillary perfusing pressure of approximately 20 cmH_2O can cause ischemic injury to the mucosa and lead to chondritis and cartilaginous necrosis. Fibrosing granulation tissue ensues, as discussed above [23]. All of these processes that injure the mucosa, promote inflammation, and trigger vascular regrowth also elevate the risk of local bleeding.

5.4 *Catastrophic Tracheostomy Tube-Related Events*

Catastrophic tracheostomy tube-related events are rare but devastating. A survey of the membership of the AAO-HNS reported 29 of 405 catastrophic events affecting children, 17 (59%) of which were fatal and 4 leading to permanent disability [7]. The most common of these events were tracheostomy-tube occlusion, decannulation, and tracheoinnominate artery fistula (TIF). Based on survey results, the authors estimate that there are approximately 1000 catastrophic tracheostomy-tube events and 500 tracheostomy-related deaths annually in the USA, affecting adults and children.

Tracheoinnominate artery fistula (TIF) is classically described as a late event occurring after the 3rd week following tracheotomy and usually within 18 months post-tracheotomy [19]. Modifiable risk factors for TIF include low tracheal incision (especially below the 3rd or 4th tracheal ring), use of a metallic tube, hyperextension of the neck, excessive movement of the tube, and excessive cuff pressure [10, 23]. A high-riding innominate artery (also known as the brachiocephalic trunk) is frequently noted [32]. Fortunately, TIF is a rare event, occurring in fewer than 1% of patients after tracheotomy [10, 23, 33]. TIF is the most commonly encountered tracheo-vascular fistula formation, but involvement of other nearby vessels has been described, including the common carotid artery, innominate vein, inferior thyroid artery, internal mammary artery, and aortic arch [19, 32]. Prior to the occurrence of devastating hemorrhage, bright red but self-limited sentinel bleeds can occur in approximately half of the patients [10, 11, 19].

Depending on the experience and training of the managing team or institution, mortality can be as high as 100% or as low as 0% [10, 32].

If the patient is of appropriate size and stability, bedside flexible tracheobronchoscopy can be performed to identify the source of tracheal bleeding [3]. In the setting of active bleeding, bronchoscopy is difficult and needs to be performed with a bronchoscope large enough to accommodate a suction channel to clear the view. Some pediatric bronchoscopes have this capacity, but the smallest tracheostomy that can accommodate the smallest pediatric flexible bronchoscope (2.8 mm) is a 3.5. Most widely available pediatric flexible bronchoscopes have an outer diameter of 5–6 mm and can only be used with pediatric tracheostomies that are 5.0 or larger. This limits the availability of the procedure for smaller patients and may prompt earlier surgical exploration if a smaller patient is clinically unstable. A consensus panel of the AAO-HNS concluded that patients with severe bleeding should undergo bronchoscopy for suspected laryngotracheal stenosis or tracheoesophageal fistula [1]. Pulsation of the tracheal wall from the innominate artery may be observed [3]. Any bright red bleeding may represent a sentinel bleed of TIF [18, 19]. In a stable patient, computed tomography-angiogram with 3D reconstruction of the neck and chest can assess the relationship of the innominate artery to the tracheal wall [3, 32].

Brisk hemorrhage can be temporized with direct pressure through multiple means. As an initial maneuver, hyperinflation of the existing tracheostomy tube cuff with minor adjustment to position the cuff over the area of bleed is often successful [34]. If bleeding persists, the tracheostomy tube can be partially withdrawn while inserting a cuffed translaryngeal (oral) endotracheal tube until its cuff is deep to the tracheostomy tube tip [3, 23, 34]. Inflating the translaryngeal tube cuff will help to reduce aspiration of blood and may further tamponade bleeding through the fistula. Finally, direct digital pressure through the stoma and anterior to the tracheostomy tube (which may still be in place) to compress the bleeding artery against the manubrium can be attempted. This is termed the Utley maneuver (Fig. 2) [19, 34]. A cardiothoracic surgery team is needed for repair of TIF. Oxygenation, transfusion of blood products, and cardiopulmonary resuscitation may be necessary while preparing for operative exploration [11, 18]. Despite successful initial surgical intervention, rebleeding associated with local infection has been described, especially with vascular reconstruction as opposed to bypass grafting [32, 35].

Prevention of TIF revolves around appropriate tracheostomy tube insertion and sizing and management of the tracheostomy tube cuff. Surveillance laryngoscopy and bronchoscopy are recommended by the ATS every 6–12 months to assess for airway pathology, detect and treat complications, assess tube size and position, and determine readiness for decannulation in children with chronic tracheostomies [14].

Because excess pressure by a tracheostomy tube cuff can erode and injure adjacent epithelium, cuff pressure needs to be carefully managed. Pressure injury by a tracheostomy tube cuff can be avoided by checking cuff pressure routinely and adjusting as necessary [1, 23]. The ideal pressure at which to inflate the tracheal tube cuff depends on patient characteristics and the design of the cuff and tube. The American Association of Respiratory Care guidelines recommend avoiding pressure >30 cmH_2O against the tracheal wall [28]. Another way to adjust cuff pressure is alternatively labeled the minimal occlusion, minimal inflation, or minimal leak technique [23, 28]. This entails inflating the cuff only as much as necessary to reduce excessive air leak around the tracheostomy tube. The patient may still have a small air leak around the cuff, but the risk of mucosal injury is reduced [23]. The effectiveness of the cuff to reduce air leakage around the tube is affected by neck

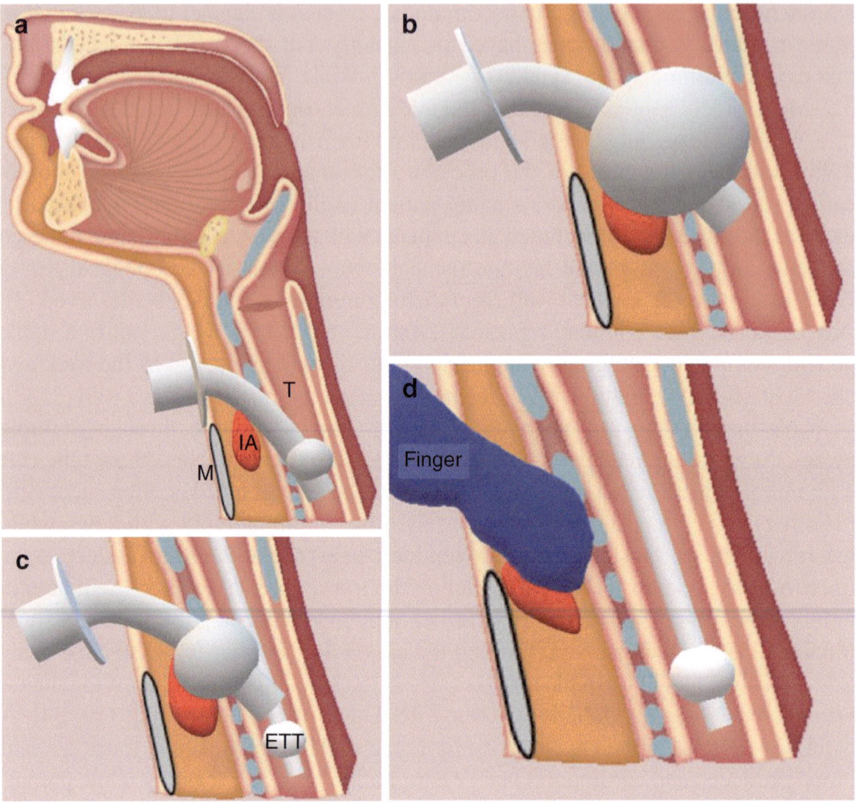

Fig. 2 Tracheoinnominate artery fistula and hemostasis maneuvers. (**a**) High-riding innominate artery (IA) adjacent to tracheostomy. M: manubrium; T: trachea. (**b**) Tracheostomy tube partially displaced with the hyperinflated tube cuff positioned to compress the innominate artery. (**c**) Translaryngeal (oral) endotracheal tube (ETT) with inflated cuff alongside the tracheostomy tube to reduce aspiration of blood. (**d**) Utley maneuver: digital compression of the innominate artery against the manubrium. Stock vector art [36] overlaid with original 3D art

and tube position. Consequently, cuff inflation and pressure may need to be adjusted for changes in patient position [28]. If greater than 30 cmH_2O is required to ensure an adequate seal, then upsizing the tube diameter may be warranted [28]. Tracheostomy tube cuffs should be deflated when a patient no longer requires mechanical ventilation [1, 28].

In summary, most episodes of bloody secretions from a tracheostomy tube are benign and resolve with conservative measures. Recognition of signs of TIF and early presentation to a facility with appropriate expertise to diagnose and manage TIF are essential for survival. Temporizing measures revolve around direct pressure to the bleeding site. Tube insertion technique, regular monitoring of established tracheostomies, and management of the tube cuff may reduce the risk of TIF.

6 Review Questions

1. Which statement below about the management of tracheostomy tube cuffs is most supported by national guidelines?
    (A) A cuffed tracheostomy tube is contraindicated for long-term use.
    (B) When using the minimal leak technique, the tracheostomy tube cuff may be inflated above manufacturer-recommended pressures if significant air leak is detected.
    (C) Inflation of tracheostomy tube cuffs prevents intermittent pulmonary aspiration in mechanically ventilated patients.
    (D) The tracheostomy tube cuff should be deflated or discontinued when a patient no longer requires mechanical ventilation.
2. Which statement below about suctioning tracheostomy tubes is most supported by national guidelines?
    (A) The largest caliber suction tube that will fit the tracheostomy tube should be used.
    (B) Tracheal wall injury should be avoided by limiting suctioning to the pre-measured length of the tracheostomy tube.
    (C) Suctioning time may exceed 5 s, as long as oxygen desaturation or other vital sign changes do not occur.
    (D) Stirring the catheter with the hand while suctioning is preferred to twirling the catheter between fingers and thumb.
3. What intervention is meant to reduce large-volume blood aspiration during tracheoinnominate artery fistula hemorrhage?
    (A) Increased positive end expiratory pressure via the mechanical ventilator
    (B) Hyperinflation of the tracheostomy tube cuff
    (C) Digital pressure on the tracheoinnominate artery fistula, or Utley maneuver
    (D) Translaryngeal (oral) endotracheal intubation with a cuffed tube

7 Answers

1. **D**. Guidelines from the American Thoracic Society, the American Academy of Otolaryngology-Head and Neck Surgery, and the American Association for Respiratory Care reached consensus on few recommendations for tracheostomy tube cuffs. Deflating or removing tracheostomy tube cuffs when mechanical ventilation is no longer needed is supported by two national guidelines. The decision to use a long-term cuff needs to be individualized. Due to the wide variety of cuffs available, manufacturer recommendations should be followed with regard to cuff inflation pressure. If excessive air leak persists despite a maximally inflated cuff, then upsizing the tracheostomy tube diameter may be

required. Intermittent aspiration has been observed in mechanically ventilated patients regardless of the inflation status of the tracheostomy tube cuff.
2. **A**. Using the largest suction tube that fits the tracheostomy tube facilitates efficient airway clearance while avoiding atelectasis and negative-pressure injury to the tracheal wall. The American Association for Respiratory Care recommendations include limiting the amount of time spent in active suctioning to less than 5 s and twirling or rotating the suction catheter between fingers and thumb instead of stirring the catheter with the hand. While limiting suction to the premeasured length of the tracheostomy tube is recommended by the American Thoracic Society, a more recent statement by the American Academy of Otolaryngology-Head and Neck Surgery did not reach consensus on the "premeasured technique."
3. **D.** Measures to apply hemostatic pressure on a bleeding tracheoinnominate artery fistula include repositioning and hyperinflating the tracheostomy tube cuff over the bleed and digital pressure. Although achieving hemostasis will incidentally reduce pulmonary aspiration of blood, the most direct measure to reduce large-volume blood aspiration is translaryngeal (oral) endotracheal intubation with a cuffed tube terminating distal to the bleeding site (Fig. 2). Positive end expiratory pressure is unlikely to have an effect on hemostasis or pulmonary aspiration.

8 Takeaway Points

1. Blood in tracheal secretions is a common complaint in patients with tracheostomy tubes.
2. Catastrophic hemorrhage can occur with tracheo-vascular fistulas, the most common of which is the tracheoinnominate artery fistula.
3. Risk factors specific to tracheoinnominate artery fistula formation include a low tracheotomy, high-riding innominate artery, neck and tube movement, and excessive cuff pressure.
4. Basic tracheostomy tube care with careful suctioning technique, meticulous cuff management, and warming and humidifying of inspired gas can reduce the risk for more common sources of tracheal bleeding.
5. Hemostatic maneuvers for tracheoinnominate artery fistula are well-described and may be lifesaving.

References

1. Mitchell RB, Hussey HM, Setzen G, Jacobs IN, Nussenbaum B, Dawson C, Brown CA, Brandt C, Deakins K, Hartnick C, Merati A. Clinical consensus statement: tracheostomy care. Otolaryngol Head Neck Surg (United States). 2013;148(1):6–20. https://doi.org/10.1177/0194599812460376.

2. Mahida JB, Asti L, Boss EF, Shah RK, Deans KJ, Minneci PC, Jatana KR. Tracheostomy placement in children younger than 2 years 30-day outcomes using the national surgical quality improvement program pediatric. JAMA Otolaryngol Head Neck Surg. 2016;142(3):241–6. https://doi.org/10.1001/jamaoto.2015.3302.
3. Watters KF. Tracheostomy in infants and children. Respir Care. 2017;62(6):799–825. https://doi.org/10.4187/respcare.05366.
4. Zhu H, Das P, Roberson DW, Jang J, Skinner ML, Paine M, Yuan J, Berry J. Hospitalizations in children with preexisting tracheostomy: a national perspective. Laryngoscope. 2015;125(2):462–8. https://doi.org/10.1002/lary.24797.
5. Edwards JD, Houtrow AJ, Lucas AR, Miller RL, Keens TG, Panitch HB, Dudley RA. Children and young adults who received tracheostomies or were initiated on long-term ventilation in PICUs. Pediatr Crit Care Med. 2016;17(8):e324–34. https://doi.org/10.1097/PCC.0000000000000844.
6. Mahadevan M, Barber C, Salkeld L, Douglas G, Mills N. Pediatric tracheotomy: 17 year review. Int J Pediatr Otorhinolaryngol. 2007;71(12):1829–35. https://doi.org/10.1016/j.ijporl.2007.08.007.
7. Das P, Zhu H, Shah RK, Roberson DW, Berry J, Skinner ML. Tracheotomy-related catastrophic events: results of a national survey. Laryngoscope. 2012;122(1):30–7. https://doi.org/10.1002/lary.22453.
8. D'Souza JN, Levi JR, Park D, Shah UK. Complications following pediatric tracheotomy. JAMA Otolaryngol Head Neck Surg. 2016;142(5):484–8. https://doi.org/10.1001/jamaoto.2016.0173.
9. Roberts J, Powell J, Begbie J, Siou G, McLarnon C, Welch A, McKean M, Thomas M, Ebdon AM, Moss S, Agbeko RS, Smith JH, Brodlie M, O'Brien C, Powell S. Pediatric tracheostomy: a large single-center experience. Laryngoscope. 2020;130(5):E375–80. https://doi.org/10.1002/lary.28160.
10. Lubianca Neto JF, Castagno OC, Schuster AK. Complications of tracheostomy in children: a systematic review. Braz J Otorhinolaryngol. 2022;88(6):882–90. https://doi.org/10.1016/j.bjorl.2020.12.006.
11. Doherty C, Neal R, English C, Cooke J, Atkinson D, Bates L, Moore J, Monks S, Bowler M, Bruce IA, Bateman N, Wyatt M, Russell J, Perkins R, McGrath BA. Multidisciplinary guidelines for the management of paediatric tracheostomy emergencies. Anaesthesia. 2018;73(11):1400–17. https://doi.org/10.1111/anae.14307.
12. Watters K, O'Neill M, Zhu H, Graham RJ, Hall M, Berry J. Two-year mortality, complications, and healthcare use in children with medicaid following tracheostomy. Laryngoscope. 2016;126(11):2611–7. https://doi.org/10.1002/lary.25972.
13. Richter A, Chen DW, Ongkasuwan J. Surveillance direct laryngoscopy and bronchoscopy in children with tracheostomies. Laryngoscope. 2015;125(10):2393–7. https://doi.org/10.1002/lary.25254.
14. Sherman JM, David S, Albamonte-Petrick SA, Chatburn RL, Fitton C, Green C, Johnston J, Lyrene RK, Myer C III, Othersen HB, Wood R, Zach M, Zander J, Zinman R. American thoracic society: care of the child with a chronic tracheostomy. Am J Respir Crit Care Med. 2000;161:297–308. https://doi.org/10.1164/ajrccm.161.1.ats1-00.
15. Carron MA, Kim SA, Sawhney R, Reidy P. Airway obstruction by granulation tissue within a fenestrated tracheotomy tube: case report. Ear Nose Throat J. 2006;85(1):54–5. https://doi.org/10.1177/014556130608500117.
16. Wilcox LJ, Weber BC, Cunningham TD, Baldassari CM. Tracheostomy complications in institutionalized children with long-term tracheostomy and ventilator dependence. Otolaryngol Head Neck Surg (United States). 2016;154(4):725–30. https://doi.org/10.1177/0194599816628486.
17. Bhatia G, Abraham V, Louis L. Tracheal granulation as a cause of unrecognized airway narrowing. J Anaesthesiol Clin Pharmacol. 2012;28(2):235–8. https://doi.org/10.4103/0970-9185.94907.
18. Batra PS, Holinger LD. Etiology and management of pediatric hemoptysis. Arch Otolaryngol Head Neck Surg. 2001;127(4):377–82. https://doi.org/10.1001/archotol.127.4.377.

19. Chauhan J, Hertzog J, Viteri S, Slamon N. Tracheoinnominate artery fistula formation in a child with long-term tracheostomy dependence. J Pediatr Intensive Care. 2019;08(02):096–9. https://doi.org/10.1055/s-0038-1672153.
20. Al-Mutairi B, Kirk V. Bacterial tracheitis in children: approach to diagnosis and treatment. Paediatr Child Health. 2004;9(1) https://doi.org/10.1093/pch/9.1.25.
21. DeBlasio D, Joseph Real F. Tracheitis. Pediatr Rev. 2020;41(9):495–7. https://doi.org/10.1542/pir.2019-0181.
22. Simon DR, Aronoff SC, del Vecchio MT. Etiologies of hemoptysis in children: a systematic review of 171 patients. Pediatr Pulmonol. 2017;52(2):255–9. https://doi.org/10.1002/ppul.23497.
23. Epstein SK. Late complications of tracheostomy. Respir Care. 2005;50(4):542–9. https://doi.org/10.1378/chest.109.1.167.
24. Gupta A, Cotton RT, Rutter MJ. Pediatric suprastomal granuloma: management and treatment. Otolaryngol Head Neck Surg. 2004;131(1):21–5. https://doi.org/10.1016/j.otohns.2004.02.036.
25. Medrek SK, Lazarus DR, Zarrin-Khameh N, Mohyuddin N, Bandi V. Obstructive post-tracheotomy granulation tissue. Am J Respir Crit Care Med. 2017;196(5):e12–3. https://doi.org/10.1164/rccm.201703-0468IM.
26. Tom LWC, Miller L, Wetmore RF, Handler SD, Potsic WP. Endoscopic assessment in children with tracheotomies. Arch Otolaryngol Head Neck Surg. 1993;119(3):321–4. https://doi.org/10.1001/archotol.1993.01880150077011.
27. Siddharth P, Mazzarella L. Granuloma associated with fenestrated tracheostomy tubes. Am J Surg. 1985;150(2):279–80. https://doi.org/10.1016/0002-9610(85)90138-2.
28. Volsko TA, Parker SW, Deakins K, Walsh BK, Fedor KL, Valika T, Ginier E, Strickland SL. AARC clinical practice guideline: management of pediatric patients with tracheostomy in the acute care setting. Respir Care. 2021;66(1):144–55. https://doi.org/10.4187/respcare.08137.
29. Elpem EH, Scott MG, Petro L, Ries MH. Pulmonary aspiration in mechanically ventilated patients with tracheostomies*. Chest. 1994;105(2):563–6. https://doi.org/10.1378/chest.105.2.563.
30. Tolep K, Leonard Getch C, Criner GJ. Swallowing dysfunction in patients receiving prolonged mechanical ventilation*. Chest. 1996;109(1):167–72. https://www.sciencedirect.com/science/article/pii/S0012369215455485
31. Schönhofer B, Barchfeld T, Haidl P, Köhler D. Scintigraphy for evaluating early aspiration after oral feeding in patients receiving prolonged ventilation via tracheostomy. Intensive Care Med. 1999;25(3):311–4. https://doi.org/10.1007/s001340050841.
32. Reger B, Neu R, Hofmann HS, Ried M. High mortality in patients with tracheoarterial fistulas: clinical experience and treatment recommendations. Interact Cardiovasc Thorac Surg. 2018;26(1):12–7. https://doi.org/10.1093/ICVTS/IVX249.
33. Peŕez-Ruiz E, Caro P, Peŕez-Frías J, Cols M, Barrio I, Torrent A, García MA, Asensio O, Pastor MD, Luna C, Torres J, Osona B, Salcedo A, Escribano A, Cortell I, Gaboli M, Valenzuela A, Aĺvarez E, Velasco R, Garciá E. Paediatric patients with a tracheostomy: a multicentre epidemiological study. Eur Respir J. 2012;40(6):1502–7. https://doi.org/10.1183/09031936.00164611.
34. Kim JH, Lee J-Y, Cho H-R, Lee JS, Ryu J-M. A 13-year-old male patient diagnosed with an anomalous arterial fistula after coming to the hospital with massive bleeding. Pediatr Emerg Med. 2015;2(2):89–92. https://doi.org/10.22470/pemj.2015.2.2.89.
35. Hung JJ, Hsu HS, Huang CS, Yang KY. Tracheoesophageal fistula and tracheo-subclavian artery fistula after tracheostomy. Eur J Cardiothorac Surg. 2007;32(4):676–8. https://doi.org/10.1016/j.ejcts.2007.06.040.
36. Captainvector. Cross-section of human mouth. Image ID 189091173. 123RF Free. 2023. https://www.123rf.com/free-vector_189091173_cross-section-of-human-mouth.html?vti=odd4vkaw5ou0rqvxe9-6-66. Accessed 8/10/2023.

A Dislodged Gastrostomy Tube

Rena Sarhangian and Kelly Fong

1 Case

A 3-year-old female with a history of hypoxic-ischemic encephalopathy, cerebral palsy, failure to thrive, and gastroesophageal reflux disease status post gastrostomy tube (G-tube) placement is brought in by her caregivers for 1 week of stomal drainage and dislodgement of her feeding tube this morning. Per her mother, about a week ago, she noticed leaking around her G-tube that consisted of a clear yellow-green fluid with some peristomal skin irritation and breakdown. The patient's pediatric gastroenterologist recommended adding water to the tube's balloon and using a barrier cream around the stoma. These interventions appeared to help initially, but then her symptoms returned. She was scheduled to follow up in gastroenterology clinic; however, this morning, the patient pulled out her G-tube and has not had her morning feeds or medications.

On physical exam, she appears well nourished although small for age. She has slightly dry mucous membranes, mild tachycardia, and brisk capillary refill. On abdominal exam, she is noted to be soft and non-tender. Her stoma has minimal clear yellow drainage, and the surrounding skin is erythematous though no induration is noted. There is a red, edematous bumpy piece of tissue on the lateral aspect of the stoma.

2 Discussion Questions

1. What is the next best step in the management of the removed G-tube?
2. What complications should be anticipated?

R. Sarhangian (✉) · K. Fong
Department of Pediatrics, UCLA Mattel Children's Hospital, Los Angeles, CA, USA
e-mail: rsarhangian@mednet.ucla.edu; kfong@mednet.ucla.edu

A. Kamzan et al. (eds.), *Children with Medical Complexity in the Emergency Department*, https://doi.org/10.1007/978-3-031-62517-6_13

3 Case Answers

1. The patient above is presenting with two issues related to her G-tube: drainage with skin irritation and dislodgement. In patients presenting with dislodgement, there are key pieces of history needed to determine appropriate management. First, it is important to determine how old the stoma is. New tubes that become dislodged within 6 weeks of initial placement require expert consultation for replacement. For mature stomas, it is important to ask the family how long the tube has been out and if they have placed anything in the stoma to keep it patent. Stomas can close in a matter of hours; therefore, it is important to maintain patency with either another feeding tube or a Foley catheter until an appropriate replacement can be obtained.
2. In patients presenting with drainage, the history and physical examination will help determine whether it is caused by the tube itself (e.g., an underinflated balloon), an anatomical issue such as granulation tissue, increased gastric pressure, or an infection. Skin surrounding the stoma should be evaluated for irritation, skin breakdown, and signs of infection. The most urgent consideration should be ensuring that the stoma does not close. If the patient's previous tube cannot be placed back into the stoma, then any other sort of tube or catheter should be placed to maintain patency. Often, skin changes are due to irritant/contact dermatitis from gastric contents. This will typically resolve with addressing the etiology of the leakage. However, if not adequately treated, patients run the risk of developing skin infections. Families should be counseled on signs and symptoms of infection and given appropriate return precautions.

4 Learning Objectives

1. Identify the causes of G-site drainage, and plan initial management steps.
2. Describe the initial management of a dislodged G-tube.
3. Understand the steps in managing a clogged G-tube.

5 Discussion

Enteral feeding tubes are one of the most common devices encountered in the care of medically complex children. They allow nutrition to be directly delivered to the stomach or small intestines. These tubes are indicated for patients unable to meet their fluid and/or caloric needs through oral intake due to a wide variety of causes. Indications are generally broken up into four broad categories: (1) feeding disorders (e.g., patients with neurological impairment), (2) dependency on fluid or nutritional supplementation (e.g., children with short gut syndrome, metabolic or renal disorders), (3) conditions where there is a physical limitation on oral intake (e.g., esophageal atresia, craniofacial anomalies), and (4) inadequate intake (e.g., inflammatory bowel disease, congenital heart disease, cystic fibrosis).

When evaluating a patient with an issue related to their enteral feeding tube, it is important to note the type of the tube (long versus low-profile gastrostomy tube), G-tube vs. GJ tube (i.e., gastrojejunostomy tube), along with the size of the tube. This is critical information for appropriate management.

Gastrostomy site tube drainage is a common complaint for which parents seek urgent evaluation in the emergency department or acute care setting. The differential is broad and includes both benign and serious conditions making it necessary to obtain a detailed history. The history should include when the drainage started, the type of fluid that is being expelled (gastric secretions, formula, etc.), color and smell of the drainage, as well as any skin changes that have occurred to the skin immediately surrounding the tube site. The most common etiologies for G-tube drainage include movement of the tube, infection, conditions that increase pressure in the stomach (such as constipation), and hypergranulation tissue (discussed below) [1].

Movement of the tube with an applied force such as inadvertent pulling can cause the stoma to enlarge and lead to subsequent leakage of gastric contents. The clear plastic disc that sits directly on the exit site also known as the external bolster should allow for 1–2 cm of movement of the tube. If the external bolster is placed either too loosely or too tightly and is not properly stabilizing the tube, peristomal leakage can result [2]. Excessive gastric acid secretion, constipation, and intestinal gas can cause increased pressure in the stomach that can result in leakage around the G-tube site. This leakage can cause skin irritation leading to erythema, itching, pain, and skin breakdown.

Management of peristomal leakage entails securing the tube and applying a skin barrier to help the surrounding skin heal. In some cases, it is necessary to remove the tube for 2–3 days to allow for constriction of the tract. A small Foley catheter can be inserted to prevent closure of the tract. It is important to note that placing a larger G-tube into the stoma site will not alleviate the problem and may potentially exacerbate the leakage by enlarging the stoma site further [3]. A proton pump inhibitor may also be indicated.

Thick green or white discharge from the stoma should raise suspicion for an infection. There may be surrounding skin erythema that is warm to the touch and painful. Fever and other systemic symptoms may also be present. If a culture of the drainage is collected, it will often show skin flora and thus has low utility. Empiric antibiotic treatment can be initiated with Keflex, Clindamycin, or Bactrim.

Granulation tissue that builds up excessively around the G-tube site can also secrete drainage. This hypergranulation tissue, unlike benign or normal granulation tissue, will be red, raised, and beefy in appearance and bleeds easily. The drainage will often be yellowish brown and appear to ooze from the tissue. Silver nitrate can be applied to the tissue for treatment. Alternatively, a topical steroid (0.5% triamcinolone cream) can be used once or twice a day until the tissue resolves [4].

Tube dislodgement will almost inevitably happen to all patients with feeding tubes. Management will depend on several factors. For gastrostomy tubes, those dislodged 6 weeks or less after initial placement are generally considered "early dislodgement," and it is appropriate for a patient to be directed to an emergency room. The team who placed the tube should be consulted for replacement as there will be concern that a false tract may be created if the tract is not mature. If a tract is mature, families may try to replace the tube at home or place a Foley or other types of catheter in the stoma to maintain patency.

For gastrojejunostomy tubes, regardless of when the tube was initially placed, replacement in the event of dislodgement must be done by a medical professional typically with either endoscopy or fluoroscopy to ensure correct placement of the jejunal portion of the tube. A gastrostomy tube should be temporarily placed to maintain patency of the stoma and facilitate medication administration if tolerated by the patient.

Lastly, a G-tube may become clogged, often because the tube is not flushed with sufficient water or medications are placed into the tube improperly. An attempt should be made to de-clog the tube with a warm-water flush. A 30 mL or 60 mL syringe is needed to avoid high pressures, and the tube is flushed with a back-and-forth motion. If this is ineffective, an enzyme solution can be used consisting of a pancreatic enzyme combined with a sodium bicarbonate tablet and 5 mL of water [5]. This solution should be allowed to dwell for 30 min and then be flushed with 30–60 mL of water. Lastly, a mechanical device, such as a long-threaded flexible plastic tool, can be inserted into the tube and used to break about any blockages.

6 Review Questions

1. Peristomal leakage can best be managed by:
   (A) Placing a larger tube into the stoma
   (B) Securing the tube properly
   (C) Removing the tube for 1 week
   (D) Starting a proton pump inhibitor

2. A patient had a GJ tube placed last week but unfortunately pulled it out an hour before presentation. The most important next step is:
   (A) Ensure that the patient is hydrated and has received any necessary meds via IV
   (B) Place a Foley catheter into the stoma site
   (C) Consult the surgical team that placed the tube for urgent evaluation
   (D) Refer the patient to GI clinic to be seen as soon as possible

3. All the following symptoms may increase a patient's risk of tube dislodgement except:
   (A) Constipation
   (B) Coughing

(C) Ambulation
(D) Vomiting

4. A patient presents with a presumed clogged tube. All the following are acceptable interventions except:

(A) Flushing with warm water
(B) Use of a stylet or guide wire to try and clear obstruction in the distal portion of the tube
(C) Instillation of pancreatic enzyme
(D) Gentle back-and-forth flushing with saline

7 Answers

1. **B**. Securing the tube properly is the best step in managing peristomal leakage. Placing a larger tube into the stoma will cause the stoma to increase and the continuation of the peristomal leakage. Removing the tube for a short period of time, such as 1–2 days, may be helpful, but removing the tube for 1 week will likely cause the tract to close.
2. **B**. Placing a Foley catheter into the stoma site is the most important next step to prevent closure of the tract. After this is done, the surgical team that placed the tube can be consulted for urgent evaluation. It is important to ensure that the patient is hydrated and has received any necessary meds via IV; however, this can occur after a Foley catheter is inserted into the stoma. A patient that had the tube removed only 1 h prior to presentation will likely be hydrated.
3. **C**. Ambulation will not increase a patient's risk of tube dislodgement. Constipation, coughing, and vomiting will increase the intra-abdominal pressure and put the patient at risk for tube dislodgement.
4. **B**. A stylet or guide wire should not be used to try to clear an obstruction. If flushing with warm water, instillation of a pancreatic enzyme, and/or gentle back-and-forth flushing with saline do not relieve the clog, a small flexible plastic tube can be used to mechanically break up the obstruction.

8 Takeaway Points

1. When a G-tube has been removed inadvertently, either another feeding tube or a Foley catheter should be used as an immediate placeholder to prevent the stoma from closing.
2. Early dislodgement of a G-tube (6 weeks or less since initial placement) requires evaluation in the emergency room or clinic by the surgical team that placed the tube to ensure that a false tract is not created.

3. Peristomal leakage from an enlarged stoma is best treated by properly securing the tube and applying a barrier cream to prevent skin irritation. Placing a larger G-tube into the stoma will only cause further enlargement and leakage.
4. Hypergranulation tissue that is red, beefy, and raised can be managed with either silver nitrate or triamcinolone cream.

References

1. Blumenstein I, Shastri YM, Stein J. Gastroenteric tube feeding: techniques, problems and solutions. World J Gastroenterol. 2014;20(26):8505–24. https://doi.org/10.3748/wjg.v20.i26.8505.
2. Wei M, Ho E, Hegde P. An overview of percutaneous endoscopic gastrostomy tube placement in the intensive care unit. J Thorac Dis. 2021;13(8):5277–96. https://doi.org/10.21037/jtd-19-3728.
3. Blinman T, Hiller D. Troubleshooting the pediatric gastrostomy. Nutr Clin Pract. 2023;38(2):240–56.
4. Hirotsu K, Kannan S, Brian Jiang SI. Treatment of hypertrophic granulation tissue: a literature review. Dermatol Surg. 2019;45(12):1507–16. https://doi.org/10.1097/DSS.0000000000002059.
5. Boeykens K, et al. Prevention and management of minor complications in percutaneous endoscopic gastrostomy. BMJ Open Gastroenterol. 2022;9(1):e000975.

A Complication of a Central Line

Yamini Sharma and Grace Sund

1 Case

A 5-year-old male with a history of gastroschisis, necrotizing enterocolitis, short gut syndrome, and total parenteral (TPN) dependence presents to the emergency department due to a central line malfunction. His mother reports that she aggressively pushed a medication through his central line, and a few hours later, the TPN was no longer infusing. She called the on-call pediatric gastroenterology physician and was advised to come to the local emergency department. Of note, her son has also had six non-bilious, non-bloody vomiting episodes and decreased oral intake over the last 2 days. While in the emergency department, a line break is visible on physical exam, and vitals are significant for a temperature of 103 °F. The patient's mom mentions that she changed the central line dressing 2 days prior to admission. He has no associated diarrhea and no change to his baseline mentation. He has had no sick contacts and no recent travel.

2 Discussion Questions

1. What is the next best step in management?
2. What complications should be anticipated?

Y. Sharma (✉) · G. Sund
Department of Pediatrics, UCLA Mattel Children's Hospital, Los Angeles, CA, USA
e-mail: YSharma@mednet.ucla.edu; GSund@mednet.ucla.edu

A. Kamzan et al. (eds.), *Children with Medical Complexity in the Emergency Department*, https://doi.org/10.1007/978-3-031-62517-6_14

3 Case Answers

1. Determine whether the line can be repaired. Draw blood cultures prior to starting broad-spectrum antibiotics. Change dressing and caps as soon as possible.
2. Patients with broken central lines and/or patients with fever in the setting of a central line are at risk for central line-associated bloodstream infections (CLABSIs).

4 Learning Objectives

1. Learn how to evaluate and manage central line breaks.
2. Understand the management of CLABSI/sepsis.
3. Recognize other common complications of central lines.

5 Discussion

The impact of effective central line management is significant. Instances of central line complications can lead to considerable adverse effects on patient well-being, including morbidity, mortality, increased length of stay, increased healthcare costs, increased antimicrobial use, and delayed recovery. The presence of indwelling catheters increases the risk of the formation of thrombi, emboli, and infection than patients with peripheral catheters by 200% [1].

There are several types of central venous catheter (CVC) devices including implanted subcutaneous infusion ports, tunneled central lines (i.e., Broviac, Hickman, dialysis), and non-tunneled central lines. An example of a non-tunneled central line is a peripherally inserted central catheter (PICC). The choice of line configuration, whether single lumen or multi-lumen, varies based on factors such as patient size, vasculature characteristics, and specific treatment requirements.

Patients with central lines are instructed to promptly seek emergency medical attention in the presence of a fever, signs and symptoms of infection, or any malfunction of the line. Such malfunctions might arise from issues like line breakage, line displacement, thrombosis, or obstruction of the catheter. Notably, this chapter will not cover the process of inserting a CVC, but will instead focus on strategies for managing risks related to line dysfunction and infection.

The rates of central line breakage are around 0.04–1.05 per 1000 catheter days in the pediatric population [2]. Repairing the line is cost effective and overall a safe and effective procedure that should be performed whenever possible. Post-procedural complications are low. The majority of studies show low or no increased risk of infection post-repair [3]. Repairing the line in the ED can decrease the number of inpatient admissions, increase patient and family satisfaction, and improve overall health outcomes [4].

The first step in a child presenting with a line break is to determine whether the line can be repaired [2]. Silastic tunneled catheters (i.e., Hickman or Broviac), whether single or double lumen, are generally repairable using a brand-specific repair kit. Repairs for PICC lines are more challenging because the length of the external catheter is much shorter at the insertion site compared to tunneled lines. If a line break occurs close to the insertion site, it may not be repairable and require full removal of the line and new insertion. If a line is repairable, it is important to consult the appropriate team (i.e., surgery or other trained staff) to assess and make the repairs as needed. Once repaired, patients are typically asked to wait a minimum of 6 h to resume usage of the line if possible. Waiting up to 24 h is ideal as this can help to ensure that the glue has fully cured (Fig. 1).

In a child with a central line who presents with fever, one set of blood cultures should be drawn from each lumen of every line. It is also recommended to obtain a peripheral blood culture if feasible. If the patient is immunocompromised, then fungal culture should also be added. When a patient has a known source of fever (e.g., pneumonia) and has had negative blood cultures during the febrile illness, they may not require blood cultures with each fever. Discussion with the primary admitting team and/or infectious disease consultants is recommended. Repeating blood cultures in patients at low risk of bacteremia may lead to false-positive blood cultures with contaminants. When CLABSI is suspected, patients should be started on broad-spectrum antibiotics within 60 min. Blood cultures should be drawn prior to the administration of antibiotics.

Other central line complications include venous thrombosis, injury to local structures, air embolism, phlebitis at the insertion site, hematoma, and catheter malposition. Catheter-related thrombosis (CRT) is defined as a venous thromboembolism (VTE) associated with the use of a CVC. CRT is on the rise due to the increased utilization of CVCs. CRT constitutes 10% of all deep venous thromboses (DVTs) in adults and 50–80% of all DVTs among children [5]. In pediatric patients, the presence of a CVC is the single most common risk factor for a VTE development. Additional risk factors for developing CRT include extended number of line days, higher number of line insertion attempts, catheter diameter relative to vein diameter, older age, and underlying thrombophilia. In pediatrics, there is a bimodal distribution with peak incidence in infancy and adolescence. Generally, CRT is asymptomatic [6]. Some studies show that femoral catheters are associated with a higher incidence of symptomatic CRT compared to upper extremity catheters [7]. Symptoms are dependent on the degree of occlusion, type of

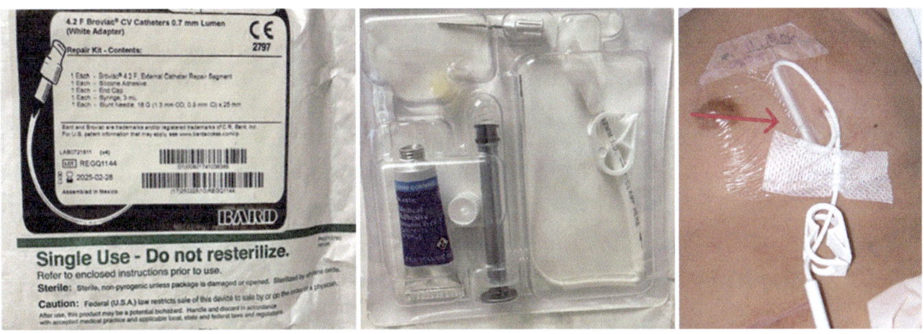

Fig. 1 Picture of what a typical repair kit looks like and a line that has been repaired

thrombus, and type of vein involved. In some cases, CRTs can present with localized pain, numbness, shoulder pain, superficial venous distension, and difficulty with aspiration or infusion [7]. It is important to consider CRT as a cause of line malfunction. One of the concerning consequences of catheter-associated thrombosis include pulmonary embolism [7]. Initial diagnostic workup should include duplex ultrasound [5]. CT venography or magnetic resonance venography (MRV) can be considered if the affected area cannot be visualized with ultrasound [5]. Of note, d-dimer has no utility in evaluating CRT patients [7].

Catheter malposition is another common but serious central line complication that can lead to perforation of the heart or great vessels. International guidelines recommend positioning the tip in the SVC or the upper part of the right atrium. Radiologically, the optimal position of the tip of the CVC should be extending ~2 vertebral bodies below the carina. Some studies have shown that subclavian and internal jugular catheters placed from the left side have higher odds of being mispositioned on the first CVC placement attempt. These CVCs can extend across the midline. Additionally, a subclavian CVC can erroneously extend through the ipsilateral jugular vein [8]. Certain changes in intrathoracic pressure and posturing can all lead to catheter mispositioning. The catheter may migrate backwards, especially in infants with chubbier necks [8]. If a catheter is malfunctioning, it is important to examine both the catheter and its skin exit site prior to obtaining imaging to assess for line breakage or wear at the clamp site. Plain radiographic views of the catheter should be acquired prior to any contrast-enhanced study [8]. The entire catheter needs to be imaged. More than one view may be needed to confirm a kink. Fluoroscopic imaging can further delineate mispositioning complications [8].

According to the US Centers for Disease Control and Prevention's (CDC) National Healthcare Safety Network (NHSN), a central line-associated bloodstream infection (CLABSI) is a laboratory-confirmed bloodstream infection that is not secondary to an infection at another body site [9, 10]. As with all healthcare-associated infections, CLABSIs are associated with high costs and consequences. According to the Agency for Healthcare Research and Quality, each infection can cost between $46,000 and $70,000 [11]. Based on CDC and Healthcare Infection Control Practices Advisory Committee (HICPAC) guidelines for prevention of catheter-related infections, most cases are considered preventable with proper aseptic techniques, consistent surveillance, and appropriate management. Compliance to an evidence-based CLABSI prevention bundle has been shown in multiple studies to have a significant impact on infection rates in various acute hospital settings [12–14].

The Association for Professionals in Infection Control and Epidemiology (APIC) emphasizes that frequent hand hygiene, appropriate use of personal protective equipment (PPE) when providers perform care, and daily catheter maintenance help prevent the risk for infection [15]. It is critical that all ports are scrubbed with institution-approved antiseptic prior to access. Providers should take into account the frequency of line access for tasks such as blood work, medication delivery, or other treatments and explore strategies to consolidate such interventions when possible. The team should discuss removing the line as soon as they are no longer necessary.

The Infusion Nurses Society provides evidence-based practice guidelines on the frequency of dressing changes based on direct observation of dressing integrity and insertion site [16]. The dressing and caps should be changed as soon as possible if the dressing has been soiled or needleless connector has presence of stagnant blood or compromised integrity. Other indications of dressing change include oozing or bleeding at the insertion site, transparent dressing in place for greater than 7 days, or nonocclusive dressing in place for over 48 h.

Patients at high risk for catheter infection include those with high stool, urine, or emesis output; patients with poor skin integrity requiring frequent dressing changes including diaphoresis; immunocompromised patients; and those with frequently clotted or occluded lines requiring alteplase. Additional factors that may put a patient at high risk for CLABSI may include parent/caregiver refusing care, "frequent flyer" patients, patients with a history of CLABSI and behavioral risk factors including playing with or biting lines, picking at skin, or scratching. When a patient experiences recurrent central line infections or malfunctions, it is essential to contemplate potential approaches for providing additional support to both the patient and their family. This can aid in devising effective strategies for enhanced line management and improved patient outcomes.

Central line catheters are considered a lifeline for many patients who are dependent on the treatments they receive. In the context of emergency departments, evaluating and addressing line-related complications and effectively managing infections are fundamental aspects of patient care (Table 1).

6 Review Questions

1. What is the recommended initial step when a patient with a central line presents to the emergency department with a malfunction?

   (A) Administer broad-spectrum antibiotics immediately
   (B) Consult the infectious disease team
   (C) Draw blood cultures from each lumen and assess line reparability
   (D) Schedule a CT scan to evaluate the line

2. What potential complications should be considered in a patient with a broken central line and fever?

   (A) Increased antimicrobial usage
   (B) Catheter-related thrombosis (CRT)
   (C) Air embolism
   (D) All of the above

3. What is the minimum waiting time before resuming the usage of a repaired central line?

   (A) 1 h
   (B) 6 h
   (C) 12 h
   (D) 24 h

Table 1 *Central line photos*

Examples of central line dressings that are clean, dry, and intact:	
Tunneled CVC with CHG disk. Loop the line up over the shoulder so it will not dangle in the diaper area 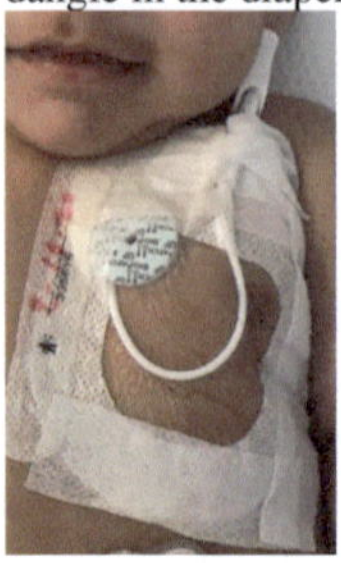	CHG gel dressing allows clear visualization of insertion site 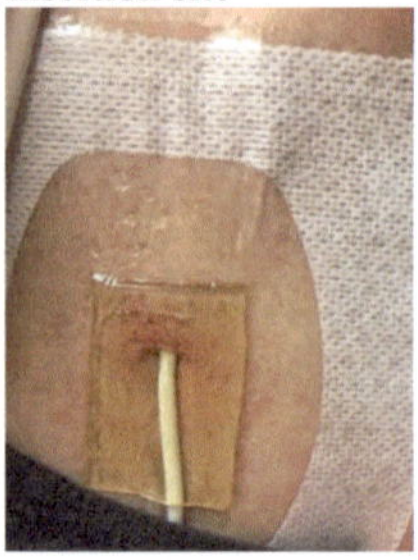
Examples of central line dressings that are problematic and must be addressed:	
Soiled dressing and integrity disrupted—do NOT reinforce, dressing must be changed immediately 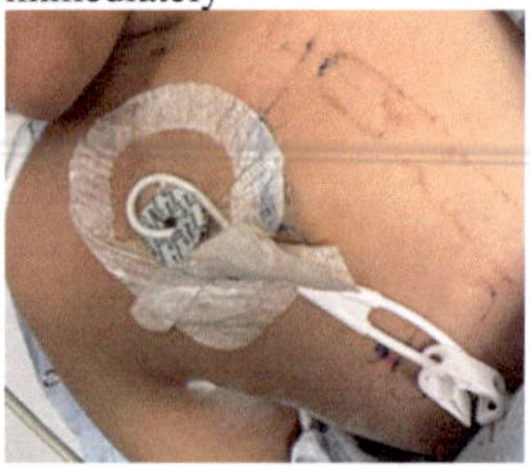	Port needle dressing with multiple reinforcements. Dressing no longer secured—dressing must be changed immediately 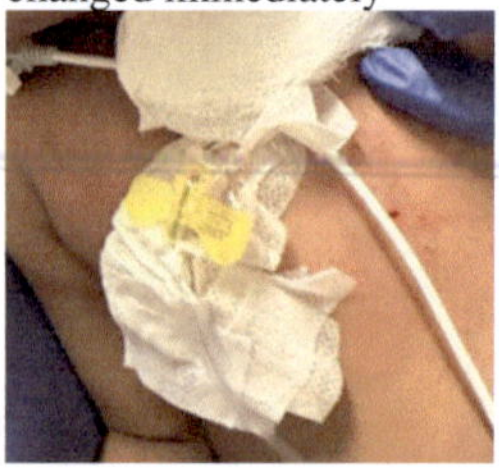
Examples of line issues that are problematic and must be addressed:	
Suture and central line cuff no longer in place, redness at insertion site—do NOT use this line; it will need to be replaced 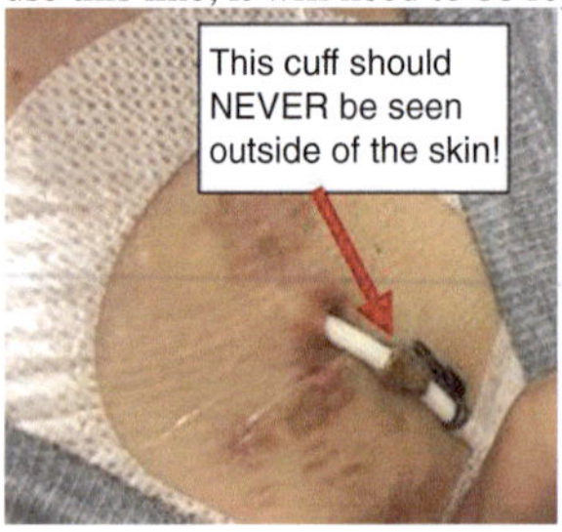	Ballooning of the inner lining of the line—do NOT use this line; it will need to be replaced 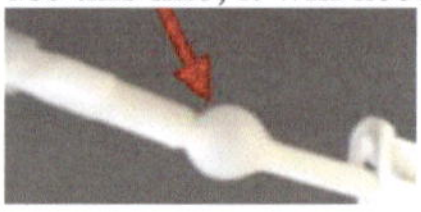 Hole/tear at the most vulnerable of the line where the thicker portion transitions to thinner—do NOT use this line; it will need to be replaced 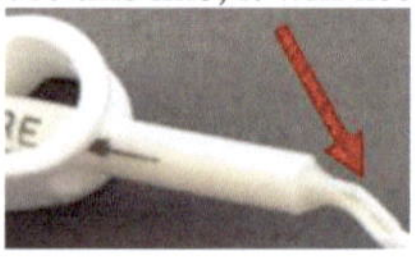

4. According to the CDC's National Healthcare Safety Network (NHSN), how is a central line-associated bloodstream infection (CLABSI) defined?
   (A) Any bloodstream infection secondary to an infection at another body site
   (B) A laboratory-confirmed bloodstream infection not secondary to an infection at another body site

(C) Any infection related to central line dressing changes
(D) A bloodstream infection with unknown origin

5. Which of the following imaging modalities can be used to detect catheter-related thrombosis?

(A) Duplex ultrasound
(B) CT venography
(C) Magnetic resonance venography (MRV)
(D) All of the above

6. When assessing catheter positioning on imaging, what is the optimal position of the tip of the CVC?

(A) Extending ~2 vertebral bodies below the carina
(B) Upper part of the right ventricle
(C) Extending ~2 vertebral bodies above the carina
(D) Lower part of the right atrium

7 Answers

1. **C**. Prior to administering antibiotics, the line must be assessed for proper function and having labs drawn. Consulting infectious disease is appropriate but not as an initial step. CT scan may be ordered to evaluate for catheter-related thrombosis, but not as an initial step.
2. **D**. Patients with central lines are instructed to promptly seek emergency medical attention in the presence of a fever, signs and symptoms of infection, or any malfunction of the line. Such malfunctions might arise from issues like line breakage, line displacement, or obstruction of the catheter. Other central line complications include venous thrombosis, injury to local structures, air embolism, phlebitis at the insertion site, hematoma, and catheter malposition.
3. **B**. Once repaired, patients are typically asked to wait a minimum of 6 h to resume usage of the line if possible. Waiting up to 24 h is ideal as this can help to ensure that the glue has fully cured.
4. **B**. According to the US Centers for Disease Control and Prevention's (CDC) National Healthcare Safety Network (NHSN), a central line-associated bloodstream infection (CLABSI) is a laboratory-confirmed bloodstream infection that is not secondary to an infection at another body site.
5. **D**. Initial diagnostic workup should include duplex ultrasound. CT venography or magnetic resonance venography (MRV) can be considered if the affected area cannot be visualized with ultrasound.
6. **A**. International guidelines recommend positioning the tip in the SVC or the upper part of the right atrium. Radiologically, the optimal position of the tip of the CVC should be extending ~2 vertebral bodies below the carina.

8 Takeaway Points

1. Patients with central lines are instructed to promptly seek emergency medical attention in the presence of fever, signs and symptoms of infection, or any malfunction of the line. Evaluating and addressing line-related complications and effectively managing infections are fundamental aspects of patient care.
2. If a catheter is malfunctioning, it is important to examine both the catheter and its exit site prior to obtaining imaging to assess for line breakage at the clamp site. Line breaks must be assessed for reparability. Once repaired, patients are asked to wait a minimum of 6 h to resume usage of the line if possible.
3. In a child with a central line who presents with fever to the emergency department, one set of blood cultures should be drawn from each lumen. Consider a peripheral blood culture in addition if feasible. If the patient is immunocompromised, then fungal culture should also be added. When CLABSI is suspected, patients should receive broad-spectrum antibiotics within 60 min.
4. Frequent hand hygiene, appropriate personal protective equipment when providers perform care, and daily catheter maintenance help prevent the risk for infection. All ports must be scrubbed with antiseptic prior to access. Aim to consolidate frequency of line access for tasks, and remove lines when they are no longer necessary.
5. High-risk factors for catheter infection include patients with high stool, urine, or emesis; those with poor skin integrity requiring frequent dressing changes; those who are immunocompromised; and patients with frequently clotted or occluded lines necessitating alteplase. Additional considerations may include patients or caregivers refusing care, "frequent flyer" patients, individuals with a history of CLABSI, and those with behavioral risk factors including playing with or biting lines, picking at skin, or scratching, which can lead to negative consequences to dressing integrity or line care.
6. Catheter-related thrombosis is frequently asymptomatic, but when symptoms are present, they can include localized pain, numbness, shoulder pain, superficial venous distension, and difficulty with aspiration or infusion. It is important to consider CRT as a cause of line malfunction.

References

1. Ball M, Singh A. Care of a Central Line. [Updated 2023 Jul 31]. In: StatPearls [Internet]. Treasure Island (FL): StatPearls Publishing; 2024 Jan-. Available from: https://www.ncbi.nlm.nih.gov/books/NBK564398/
2. Lundgren IS, Zhou C, Malone FR, McAfee NG, Gantt S, Zerr DM. Central venous catheter repair is associated with an increased risk of bacteremia and central line-associated bloodstream infection in pediatric patients. Pediatr Infect Dis J. 2012;31(4):337–40.
3. Taroc AM, Sullivan E. Identifying odds of bloodstream infection in repaired silastic central venous catheters in a pediatric population. Br J Nurs. 2023;32(7):S32–6. https://doi.org/10.12968/bjon.2023.32.7.S32

4. Wallace-Shaw K, Adigun A, Mohandas A, Costa A, Markley M, Duro D. A multidisciplinary approach and development of an algorithm for timely repair of central venous access in pediatric patients. Cureus. 2022;14(3):e23355. https://doi.org/10.7759/cureus.23355
5. Citla Sridhar D, Abou-Ismail MY, Ahuja SP. Central venous catheter-related thrombosis in children and adults. Thromb Res. 2020;187:103–12. https://doi.org/10.1016/j.thromres.2020.01.017
6. Gray BW, Gonzalez R, Warrier KS, Stephens LA, Drongowski RA, Pipe SW, Mychaliska GB. Characterization of central venous catheter-associated deep venous thrombosis in infants. J Pediatr Surg. 2012;47(6):1159–66. https://doi.org/10.1016/j.jpedsurg.2012.03.043
7. Wall C, Moore J, Thachil J. Catheter-related thrombosis: a practical approach. J Intensive Care Soc. 2016;17(2):160–7. https://doi.org/10.1177/1751143715618683
8. Barnacle, A., Arthurs, O.J., Roebuck, D. et al. Malfunctioning central venous catheters in children: a diagnostic approach. Pediatr Radiol 38, 363–378 (2008). https://doi.org/10.1007/s00247-007-0610-2
9. US Centers for Disease Control and Prevention, National Healthcare Safety Network. Device-Associated (DA) Module. Protocol and Instructions: Central Line-Associated Bloodstream Infection (CLABSI) Event. Jan 2012.
10. Centers for Disease Control and Prevention. Guidelines for the prevention of intravascular catheter-related infections (2011, revised 2017). Retrieved from https://www.cdc.gov/infectioncontrol/guidelines/bsi/recommendations.html
11. Agency for Healthcare Research and Quality. Estimating the additional hospital inpatient cost and mortality associated with selected hospital-acquired infections, November 2017. Retrieved from https://www.ahrq.gov/sites/default/files/publications2/files/hac-cost-report2017.pdf
12. Lee KH, Cho NH, Jeong SJ, Kim MN, Han SH, Song YG. Effect of central line bundle compliance on central line-associated bloodstream infections. Yonsei Med J. 2018;59(3):376–82.
13. O'Grady NP, Alexander M, Burns LA, Dellinger EP, Garland J, Heard SO, Lipsett PA, Masur H, Mermel LA, Pearson ML, Raad II, Randolph AG, Rupp ME, Saint S. Healthcare Infection Control Practices Advisory Committee (HICPAC). Guidelines for the prevention of intravascular catheter-related infections. Clin Infect Dis. 2011;52(9):e162–93.
14. Children's Hospitals Solutions for Patient Safety. Solutions for patient safety prevention bundles. Available at www.solutionsforpatientsafety.org/for-hospitals/hospital-resources/. Accessed September 8, 2023
15. Association of Professionals in Infection Control and Epidemiology (APIC). Guide to preventing central line-associated bloodstream infections, (2015). Retrieved March 29, 2022 from http://apic.org/Resource_/TinyMceFileManager/2015/APIC_CLABSI_WEB.pdf
16. Gorski HL, Hagle ME, Broadhurst D, Clare S, Kleidon T, Meyer BM, Nickel B, Rowley S, Sharpe E, Alexander M. Infusion therapy standards of practice, 8th edition. J Infus Nurs. 2021;44(1S):S1–S224.

A Complication of Bladder Reconstruction

Elizabeth Mannino Avila, George Chiang, and Julia Beauchamp Walters

1 Case

A 13-year-old male with a history of myelomeningocele, ventriculoperitoneal (VP) shunt, and neurogenic bowel and bladder presents with 1 day of fever, nausea, and abdominal pain. Four months prior to presentation, he underwent complex urological surgery including bladder neck reconstruction, small bowel resection, augmentation cystoplasty, double-Monti procedure in a Mitrofanoff fashion, suprapubic catheter (SPC) placement, and laparoscopic-assisted Malone antegrade colonic enema (ACE). He performs bladder irrigations twice a day and clean intermittent catheterization every 3 h through the Mitrofanoff. Additionally, he flushes the ACE daily with tap water mixed with baby shampoo. An indwelling catheter is left in place overnight through the Mitrofanoff and the ACE (which is standard practice during the first postoperative year). He denies problems with catheterization of either the Mitrofanoff or the ACE. He denies change in urine color or smell. His medications include oxybutynin and polyethylene glycol. His other surgical history

---

E. M. Avila
Department of Pediatric Hospital Medicine, Rady Children's Hospital San Diego, University of California, San Diego, CA, USA
e-mail: emavila@rchsd.org

G. Chiang
Department of Urology, RCHSD Chief of Pediatric Urology, University of California, San Diego, CA, USA
e-mail: gchiang@rchsd.org

J. B. Walters (✉)
Department of Pediatric Hospital Medicine, Rady Children's Hospital San Diego, Interim Co-Chief Pediatric Hospital Medicine, University of California, San Diego, CA, USA
e-mail: jbeauchamp@rchsd.org

A. Kamzan et al. (eds.), *Children with Medical Complexity in the Emergency Department*, https://doi.org/10.1007/978-3-031-62517-6_15

includes myelomeningocele repair and VP shunt placement as an infant and a number of orthopedic procedures.

On exam, his vital signs are as follows: T 100.9 °F, P 154, RR 40, BP 147/75, Sat 91% RA, 99% 3L via NC, and GCS 15. He is conversant and able to answer questions, but he is ill-appearing. His exam is notable for intact sensory level just above the umbilicus. His abdomen is distended with hypoactive bowel sounds and diffuse tenderness to palpation. The Mitrofanoff and ACE are without surrounding erythema or bleeding.

Laboratory studies are notable for an elevated white blood cell count of 17.5×10^3 cells/μL, with normal C-reactive protein and lactic acid. A basic metabolic panel is unremarkable aside from elevated creatinine to 0.9 mg/dL. His urinalysis is notable for blood, protein, 3+ LE, 1402 WBC/μL, and rare bacteria. A non-contrast CT scan of the abdomen and pelvis reveals moderate ascites in all four quadrants but no intra-abdominal abscess. The surgically reconstructed neobladder is notable for irregularly thickened walls. His VP shunt catheter is in place.

2 Discussion Questions

1. What postoperative complications might explain the imaging findings?
2. What is the next best step in management?

3 Case Answers

1. Given the history of the bladder augmentation, life-threatening bladder rupture must be ruled out. Bladder perforation can occur as both an early and late complication of cystoplasty.
2. A cystogram, via either computerized tomography (CT) or fluoroscopy, is the imaging study of choice to evaluate for bladder perforation.

4 Learning Objectives

1. Understand the indications for continent catheterizable channels. (Mitrofanoff/Monti) and role of bladder reconstruction (augmentation cystoplasty).
2. Review the basic anatomy of Mitrofanoff/Monti procedures and maintenance care.
3. Describe common complications in both the postoperative period and long-term setting.

5 Discussion

Children with congenital malformations, such as meningomyelocele (spina bifida), cloacal exstrophy, and posterior urethral valves, often suffer from bladder dysfunction, commonly referred to as neurogenic bladder. Children with severe brain injury or spinal cord disease may also suffer from neurogenic bladder. As children with neurogenic bladder mature, urinary continence becomes an important healthcare goal. Continent catheterizable channels (CCCs), such as the Mitrofanoff, first described by the surgeon Paul Mitrofanoff in 1980 as a "trans-appendicular continent cystostomy," offer a solution. The Mitrofanoff procedure utilizes the appendix, with intact mesenteric blood supply, to create a channel from the bladder to the skin of the abdomen (Fig. 1). The surgical technique involves creation of an anti-refluxing submucosal tunnel at the bladder insertion [1]. A positive pressure gradient is created between the channel lumen and the bladder, thereby preventing urine leakage and allowing for clean intermittent catheterization (CIC) for bladder emptying. The bladder must be capable of holding a large volume of urine at low pressure for the CCC to function as a continent channel. When bladder pressure is high or of low capacitance, bladder augmentation or cystoplasty is necessary [2]. The Mitrofanoff technique consists of:

1. A continent catheterizable channel (CCC)
2. An easy-to-access stoma, e.g., at the umbilicus
3. A low-pressure bladder with good capacity

In addition to the appendix, other structures such as ureters, fallopian tubes, and transverse ileum (Monti or Yang Monti) have been used to create CCC. At present, intestinal tissue is most commonly used. The channel may be inserted into various locations in the bladder or into part of the reconstructed bladder and then connected

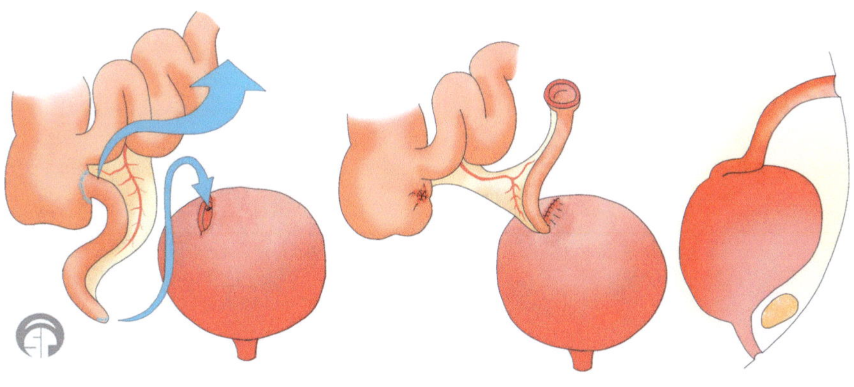

Fig. 1 Mitrofanoff illustration. Appendix is repositioned into the bladder and skin while maintaining mesenteric blood supply. File:Mitrofanoff.jpg. (2020, October 16). *Wikimedia Commons*. Retrieved 19:56, July 20, 2023 from https://commons.wikimedia.org/w/index.php?title=File:Mitrofanoff.jpg&oldid=491675479

to the abdominal wall. The stoma on the abdominal wall is often placed either in the umbilicus or in the lower abdomen for cosmesis and ease of self-catheterization (Fig. 2). Many children undergoing CCC creation, including the patient in our case presentation, have small, poorly compliant neurogenic bladders that must be augmented in order to create an appropriate low-pressure system. Generally, ileum is used, although care must be taken not to risk long-term vitamin B12 deficiency, as B12 is absorbed in the ileum. In addition, augmentation can be performed utilizing colon or stomach; however, ileum or sigmoid reaches the pelvis easiest for augmentation purposes. Any enteric segment used can predispose to metabolic abnormalities or nutrient deficiencies. The choice of tissue for CCC as well as bladder cystoplasty is determined by patient factors including history of prior bowel surgeries, length of channel required, and if concomitant ACE will be performed. Like CCC, ACE offers the patient more autonomy, with increased control of bowel function. If concomitant ACE is performed, the appendix is typically used for creation of the antegrade channel into the cecum.

There are complications related to creation of CCC and bladder reconstruction in both the immediate postoperative period and long term. As with any major abdominal surgery, risks of serious complications in the postoperative period include bleeding, bowel obstruction, ileus, infection, or anastomotic leak [3]. The most common complications of CCC include stenosis or stricture of the channel [4], bladder stones, incontinence, and urinary tract infections (UTIs). Diagnosis of UTI in patients with neurogenic bladder is often challenging as asymptomatic chronic bacteriuria is common. However, urinary tract infections are common, even using the diagnostic criteria of symptoms (e.g., fever, malaise, discomfort) and urine studies. Patients who do not fully empty their bladders have higher rates of UTI, as well as higher rates of bladder stones [5]. The most frequently reported long-term complications are channel stenosis, incontinence, and need for surgical revision [3]. Other less common complications include perforation, prolapse, kinking, pouch formation within the channel, and false passage of a catheter [2]. Late complications may also occur, including bowel strictures, leaks, and hernias. When bladder

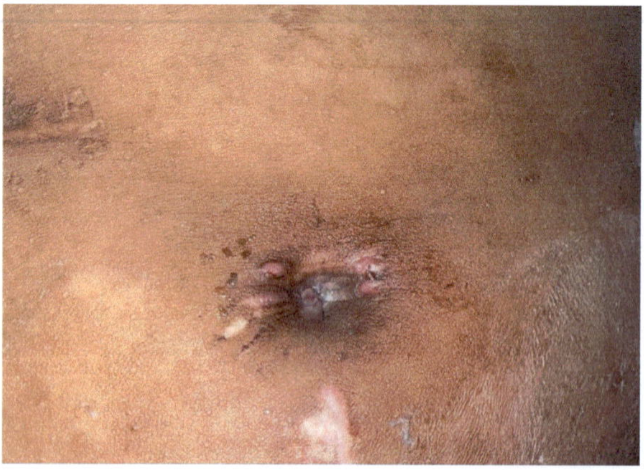

Fig. 2 Mitrofanoff channel at umbilicus

augmentation is also performed during the procedure, major complications include bladder perforation and fistula formation [6, 7]. All patients with augmented bladders need to irrigate the neobladder with normal saline at least once daily for the rest of their lives. The volume of saline is expected to increase over time as the bladder increases in size. Bladder perforation can occur at any time and is thought to be associated with persistently elevated bladder pressure and noncompliance with clean intermittent catheterization or irrigation protocols. Many patients require intermittent botulinum toxin injections to decrease bladder spasm and improve bladder compliance. Bladder perforation has a reported incidence ranging from 0.8% to 13% [7–9]. Other complications of bladder augmentation include hyperchloremic metabolic acidosis which is thought to be mediated by increased absorption of aluminum chloride relative to secretion of sodium bicarbonate by the enteric epithelium. While the hope is that creation of the CCC and bladder augmentation will alleviate upper urinary tract disease, kidney disease can worsen despite these procedures. Table 1 provides a summary of surgical procedures described with associated benefits and potential complications.

For our patient, the differential diagnosis of ascites or non-physiologic amounts of intraperitoneal free fluid is broad and can be divided by nature of the fluid content as either transudate or exudate. The differential diagnosis for transudates includes disorders associated with low oncotic pressure (such as nephrotic syndrome and protein-losing enteropathy) and those with increased intravascular pressure (such as congestive heart failure and portal hypertension). Exudates are more commonly seen with infections (such as UTI, appendicitis, infectious colitis, sexually transmitted infections/pelvic inflammatory disease), inflammatory disorders (such as Crohn's, ulcerative colitis, and lupus), and neoplasms (lymphoma, hepatoblastoma). In our patient, the differential diagnosis is further compounded by the presence of a VP shunt and extensive prior surgeries. Given the VP shunt, the clinician must consider the possibility of a peritoneal cerebrospinal (CSF) pseudocyst, or "CSF-oma," caused by either a low-grade shunt infection, elevated CSF protein, or peritoneal adhesions. Additionally, the clinician must be aware of the potential for extension from infected intraperitoneal fluid into the CSF. Finally, given the bladder cystoplasty, bladder perforation must be ruled out as it is associated with high morbidity and mortality. Additional postoperative considerations include leakage at other surgical anastomosis sites, or through a perforation incurred during intermittent catheterization.

For our patient, a CT cystogram revealed extravasation of contrast from the bladder into the peritoneum along the posterior aspect of the neobladder (Fig. 3). The patient was taken to the operating room where the peritoneum was irrigated, neobladder perforation repaired, and a suprapubic catheter (SPC) placed. Both Mitrofanoff and SPC were left to drainage. A urine culture was positive for *E. coli* and *Klebsiella pneumoniae*, while the initial blood culture grew *E. coli* only. He was stabilized in the pediatric intensive care unit; however, despite early initiation of broad-spectrum antibiotics, his course was complicated by the development of intraperitoneal abscesses that required drainage and externalization of the VP shunt. Abscess cultures were positive for *E. coli* and *Klebsiella*, but CSF culture revealed no

Table 1 Summary of common urological procedures for patients with neurogenic bladder

Procedure	Description	Benefits	Drawbacks/ complications
Vesicostomy	Continuous bladder drainage through cutaneous channel	No need for CIC (unless stenosis occurs)	Incontinence
Continent catheterizable channel (a) Mitrofanoff (b) Yang Monti (c) Double Monti *Choice of CCC is determined by the need for concomitant M-ACE and length of channel required	(a) Use of appendix (b) Use of ileal segment (c) Use of two ileal segments	Continence, autonomy, improved personal hygiene and quality of life	Need for CIC Complications: 1. Leakage (incontinence) 2. Stricture 3. Infection 4. Prolapse 5. Perforation (if patient also has an augmentation) 6. Mucus production 7. Need for revision
Bladder augmentation/ cystoplasty	Bladder augmentation using bowel segment, most common ileocystoplasty	Improved bladder capacitance and compliance, preservation of renal function, improvement in VUR/ hydronephrosis	Early complications: 1. Leak/perforation 2. Small bowel obstruction (SBO) 3. Infection of VP shunt if present Late complications: 1. Leak/perforation 2. Bladder stones 3. SBO 4. Fistula 5. Recurrent UTI 6. Chronic kidney disease 7. Bladder adenocarcinoma 8. Metabolic alkalosis 9. Hematuria-dysuria syndrome
MACE (Malone Antegrade Continence Enema)	Attachment of appendix to cecum to deliver enemas to treat chronic constipation secondary to neurogenic bowel	Autonomy, improved personal hygiene and quality of life	Complications: 1. Stomal stenosis 2. Leakage through the stoma 3. Prolapse 4. Difficulty/pain with stoma catheterization

growth. The externalized VP shunt was relocated into the right atrium by neurosurgery. A follow-up voiding cystourethrogram performed 3 weeks after surgical repair did not reveal residual leak of the neobladder. He was discharged home with drainage catheters in place for both the SPC and Mitrofanoff, to be removed in outpatient follow-up.

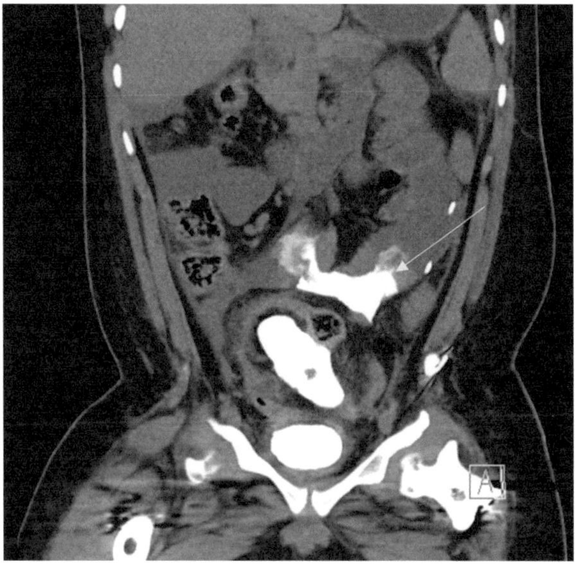

Fig. 3 CT image of contrast extravasation (yellow arrow)

6 Review Questions

1. Which three components are needed for a Mitrofanoff or similar procedure to be successful?
   (A) A continent urethra, low-pressure bladder, and an easy-to-access stoma
   (B) A continent catheterizable channel, low-pressure bladder, and an easy-to-access stoma
   (C) A continent catheterizable channel, high-pressure bladder, and suprapubic stoma
   (D) A continent urethra, high-pressure bladder, and easy-to-access stoma
2. Which of these is *not* a common complication of a CCC?
   (A) Channel stenosis
   (B) Bladder stones
   (C) Perforation
   (D) UTI
3. What is the best study to evaluate for bladder perforation?
   (A) MRI abdomen/pelvis with and without contrast
   (B) Cystogram
   (C) Renal and bladder ultrasound with Doppler
   (D) FAST exam

7 Answers

1. **B.** For a Mitrofanoff to be successful, one needs a continent catheterizable channel, low-pressure bladder, and easy-to-access stoma. For this reason, many of the children who undergo a Mitrofanoff or similar procedure must also undergo bladder augmentation, which increases the risk of bladder rupture. The urethra does not have to remain patent, although typically it is left so. As the idea of a Mitrofanoff is to allow for some independence as well as continence, the stoma must be in a location that is aesthetically pleasing and easy to access for the patient to self-catheterize.
2. **C.** The most common complications of a CCC are channel stenosis, bladder stones, and UTI. Other common complications include incontinence. Perforation, while a very serious complication, is less common, as are false tracks, bladder/bowel leak, fistula formation, bowel obstruction, and kinking.
3. **B.** A CT or fluoroscopic cystogram is the best study to evaluate for bladder perforation even though other modalities (for example, ultrasound or MRI) may identify the non-physiologic free fluid.

8 Takeaway Points

1. Bladder rupture is a serious complication of bladder augmentation and should be included in the differential diagnosis of patients with a history of bladder augmentation and Mitrofanoff presenting with free peritoneal fluid and shock.
2. Maintenance of Mitrofanoff and bladder augmentation includes regular intermittent catheterization and bladder irrigation for life.
3. A low-pressure system is required for the CCC to maintain continence; hence, some patients may require botulinum toxin injections of the neobladder.
4. The clinician must be aware of both the emergent surgical complications and the long-term complications associated with bladder augmentation and CCC procedures.

References

1. Mitrofanoff P. [Trans-appendicular continent cystostomy in the management of the neurogenic bladder]. Chir Pediatr. 1980;21(4):297–305. Cystostomie continente trans-appendiculaire dans le traitement des vessies neurologiques
2. Farrugia MK, Malone PS. Educational article: the Mitrofanoff procedure. J Pediatr Urol. 2010;6(4):330–7. https://doi.org/10.1016/j.jpurol.2010.01.015.
3. Veeratterapillay R, Morton H, Thorpe AC, Harding C. Reconstructing the lower urinary tract: the Mitrofanoff principle. Indian J Urol. 2013;29(4):316–21. https://doi.org/10.4103/0970-1591.120113.

4. Abdelhalim A, Omar H, Edwan M, et al. Reoperation for channel complications in children with continent cutaneous catheterizable channels: the test of time. Urology. 2022;159:196–202. https://doi.org/10.1016/j.urology.2021.08.015.
5. Iqbal N, Syed OZ, Bukhari AH, et al. Utility of Mitrofanoff as bladder draining tool: a single center experience in pediatric patients. Turk J Urol. 2019;45(1):42–7. https://doi.org/10.5152/tud.2018.86836.
6. Husmann DA. Lessons learned from the management of adults who have undergone augmentation for spina bifida and bladder exstrophy: Incidence and management of the non-lethal complications of bladder augmentation. Int J Urol. 2018;25(2):94–101. https://doi.org/10.1111/iju.13417.
7. Husmann DA. Mortality following augmentation cystoplasty: a transitional urologist's viewpoint. J Pediatr Urol. 2017;13(4):358–64. https://doi.org/10.1016/j.jpurol.2017.05.008.
8. DeFoor W, Tackett L, Minevich E, Wacksman J, Sheldon C. Risk factors for spontaneous bladder perforation after augmentation cystoplasty. Urology. 2003;62(4):737–41. https://doi.org/10.1016/s0090-4295(03)00678-2.
9. Breen M, Phelps A, Estrada C, Chow JS. The role of imaging in pediatric bladder augmentation. Pediatr Radiol. 2015;45(10):1440–7. https://doi.org/10.1007/s00247-015-3349-1.

Further Reading

Farrugia MK, Malone PS. Educational article: the Mitrofanoff procedure. J Pediatr Urol. 2010;6:330–7.

Husmann DA. Lessons learned from the management of adults who have undergone augmentation for spina bifida and bladder exstrophy: Incidence and management of the non-lethal complications of bladder augmentation. Int J Urol. 2018;25(2):94–101. https://doi.org/10.1111/iju.13417. Epub 2017 Aug 3

Merriman LS, Arlen AM, Kirsch AJ, Leong T, Smith E. Does augmentation cystoplasty with continent reconstruction at a young age increase the risk of complications or secondary surgeries? J Pediatr Urol. 2015;11:41.e1–5.

A Child with a Ventriculoperitoneal Shunt and Fever

Jasen Liu, Vivian Lin, Kristina Adachi, and Anthony Wang

1 Case

A 6-year-old boy with myelomeningocele status post repair as an infant, hydrocephalus status post ventriculoperitoneal (VP) shunt placement at age 1, with most recent revision about 3 months ago, and neurogenic bladder requiring intermittent catheterization presents to the emergency department for 1 day of fever, vomiting, headache, and abdominal pain. The fever started last night after he came back from school, with a maximum measured axillary temperature of 102 °F. His emesis is non-bloody and nonbilious, and he has been unable to keep any food or fluids down. The abdominal pain is described as a diffuse achy pain without radiation. He is unable to describe the headache. The fevers, headache, and abdominal pain respond briefly to acetaminophen. There is no associated runny nose, cough, sore throat, diarrhea, or rash. The patient does have baseline constipation, and his last bowel movement was 2 days ago and noted as normal. The patient's urine output has decreased, but his parents have not noticed significant changes to the color or smell of the urine. He is more tired than usual per his parents.

In the emergency department, his vital signs include temperature of 101.8 °F, heart rate of 144 beats/min, blood pressure of 110/69 mmHg, respiratory rate of 32 breaths/min, and oxygen saturation of 98%. On exam, he appears uncomfortable with dry mucous membranes. His VP shunt is palpable over the right temporal area coursing down right neck without any overlying erythema, edema, or tenderness. His abdomen is tender to palpation diffusely without peritonitic signs.

J. Liu (✉) · V. Lin · K. Adachi
Department of Pediatrics, UCLA, Los Angeles, CA, USA
e-mail: jasenliu@mednet.ucla.edu; vivianlin@mednet.ucla.edu; kadachi@mednet.ucla.edu

A. Wang
Department of Neurosurgery, UCLA, Los Angeles, CA, USA
e-mail: acwang@mednet.ucla.edu

A. Kamzan et al. (eds.), *Children with Medical Complexity in the Emergency Department*, https://doi.org/10.1007/978-3-031-62517-6_16

2 Discussion Questions

1. What is your differential diagnosis?
2. What is the next best step in diagnosis?

3 Case Answers

1. This patient's presentation including a fever, abdominal pain, headache, and fatigue may be consistent with a shunt infection, viral syndrome, urinary tract infection, or appendicitis.
2. The next best step in diagnosis includes a rapid-sequence MRI (CT head without contrast if MRI unavailable), X-ray shunt series, and a lumbar puncture/shunt tap in addition to more standard workup for the other diagnoses in consideration.

4 Learning Objectives

1. Understand the basic components of a ventricular shunt
2. Describe the most common complications of ventricular shunts
3. Understand the initial management of ventricular shunt complications

5 Discussion

Ventricular shunts are commonly placed in children with intracranial pathologies that lead to imbalances in cerebral spinal fluid (CSF) flow homeostasis, in order to manage a resultant increase in intracranial pressure. In the pediatric population, hydrocephalus is the most common indication for ventricular shunt placement and is most commonly associated with intraventricular hemorrhage (a common complication of prematurity), myelomeningocele, or brain tumors. Other less common causes include congenital aqueduct stenosis, infections of the central nervous system, and head injuries [1].

Modern ventricular shunts are comprised of three basic components: a ventricular catheter, a pressure-sensitive flow-limiting valve, and distal tubing. The proximal ventricular catheter is situated within (most commonly) one of the lateral ventricles, as the name suggests. The preferred location for distal catheter placement is in the peritoneum (ventriculoperitoneal shunt), due to superior long-term patency and lower complication rate.

The diversion of CSF is achieved when the intracranial pressure rises to a level above a pressure threshold defined by the shunt valve. Valves are typically either fixed pressure or externally programmable [2]. Once the intraventricular CSF pressure rises higher than the set threshold, the valve opens to allow drainage of CSF.

Rarely, the peritoneum may be unsuitable for distal shunt placement, such as in children having had multiple abdominal surgeries and resultant scarring or with an active abdominal infection. Common alternative sites of distal shunt placement include the pleural cavity (ventriculopleural shunt) or the distal superior vena cava (ventriculoatrial shunt).

For the purposes of this review, focus and attention will be paid to ventriculoperitoneal (VP) shunts, as they are the most frequently encountered in practice.

5.1 *Noninfectious Complications*

Complications from VP shunts are common, with rates of shunt failure approaching 40–50% within the first 2 years after placement [3]. Complications can broadly be categorized as noninfectious vs. infectious in origin.

Noninfectious complications include shunt obstruction, fracture or disconnection along the shunt system, migration or misplacement of a component of the shunt system (most commonly the distal catheter), and CSF over-drainage.

VP shunt obstructions are the most common mechanical complication of shunts and tend to occur within the first year of placement [4]. Obstruction can happen at any level along the shunt path, but is most commonly seen at the ventricular catheter. Growth of brain parenchyma or choroid plexus into the shunt lumen, or buildup of cellular debris, is thought to be the most common cause of proximal shunt obstruction. Less commonly, obstruction can occur within the valve from tissue debris or blood clots after recent shunt insertion or revision.

Misplacement of either the intracranial or the distal portion of the shunt system must be considered after recent shunt insertion or revision. Migration of the ventricular catheter is rare, though changes in the brain with either decompression or growth of the patient can have the same effect. Migration of the distal shunt catheter is far more common and can present in myriad ways. Some better recognized scenarios include erosion into bowel, bladder, or uterus; migration out of the peritoneal cavity into the abdominal fat; and migration into the venous system. Disconnection or fracture, on the other hand, is usually a late complication and occurs after a component of the shunt becomes adherent and fixated, and either growth or movement of the patient then stretches the shunt system [5]. The most common site of fracture is along the neck, in the setting of calcifications fixating the distal shunt tubing at this site.

Early and late complications of CSF over-drainage are typical. Excessive drainage of CSF is often marked by low-pressure or positional "spinal" headaches. In children with high brain compliance, CSF over-drainage may lead to a rapid decrease in ventricular size, collapse of the brain, and, potentially, development of subdural bleeding. This complication is most often seen within days to weeks of VP shunt placement. Conversely, slit-ventricle syndrome is a late complication related to chronic over-drainage marked by chronic headaches no longer affected by CSF pressure alteration or shunt manipulation [5].

5.1.1 Risk Factors

Younger age at the time of shunt placement represents a significant risk factor for failure. Other factors include recent shunt revision within 6 months, cerebral nervous system (CNS) or shunt infection, and number of prior shunt operations [3].

5.1.2 Signs and Symptoms

Clinical manifestations of mechanical shunt failures can include irritability, nausea, vomiting, headache, progressive lethargy, poor feeding, new seizure or changes in seizure pattern, swelling along shunt site/tubing, or vision changes. In infants, disproportionately increasing head circumference, bulging fontanelles, altered mental status, papilledema, or cranial nerve palsies may be noted.

5.1.3 Workup and Diagnosis

- Rapid-sequence magnetic resonance imaging (MRI) of the brain (or non-contrast CT, if MRI is unavailable) is performed to evaluate for ventricular dilation, as well as to examine for secondary signs of hydrocephalus such as trans-ependymal CSF migration. X-ray imaging along the length of the shunt (also known as a shunt series) is also part of the standard initial workup for shunt malfunction, as it can reveal complications such as shunt system discontinuity or migration. Once these and other systemic evaluations are complete, a pediatric neurosurgeon should be urgently consulted to evaluate any findings suggesting shunt malfunction.

5.1.4 Management

Shunt malfunctions require urgent neurosurgical intervention for correction and management, as replacement of the failing shunt component(s) is the definitive treatment.

5.2 *CSF Shunt Infections*

Shunt infections comprise the other large portion of VP shunt complications and are a major cause of morbidity and hospitalization in patients with VP shunts. For the purposes of this section, VP shunt infections are considered infections that involve the CSF in patients with VP shunts (i.e., device-related meningitis or ventriculitis). As the signs and symptoms of VP shunt infections can be nonspecific and subtle, and the morbidity associated with infections can be severe, providers need to have a high index of suspicion for infection when approaching patients with VP shunts.

5.2.1 Epidemiology and Timing

Rates of shunt infections range among different sources, but incidences in the 4–17% range are often cited [6]. The timing of shunt infections, however, is well-established. Shunt infections are most commonly an early complication of VP shunt placement. Most infections are seen within the first 2 months of placement (60–70%), with nearly 90% of cases seen within the first 6 months [6].

5.2.2 Risk Factors

While various risk factors have been noted in many studies, the age of the patient at the time of VP shunt placement remains one of the most consistent [6]. Infection rates are higher in children compared to adults, and patients under 6 months of age at the time of placement are noted to have the highest rates. A history of prematurity is also known to increase the risk of infections. Other factors that are often noted include etiology of hydrocephalus (with intraventricular hemorrhage and myelomeningocele representing the highest risks), history of prior infections or revisions, and poor postoperative wound healing.

5.2.3 Pathogenesis

Due to the high rates of infections seen early following surgical placement, the pathogenesis of the majority of infections is thought to be related to contamination of either the surgical site or the shunt itself at the time of placement [7]. Other mechanisms include (1) infections that start at the distal catheter end that then spread retrograde to the CSF, often as the result of the development of an infected pseudocyst or perforation of an abdominal viscus organ; (2) infections that spread from the skin, as in the case of cellulitis adjacent to hardware; (3) direct inoculation from the insertion of a needle into a shunt reservoir; or (4) hematogenous spread of bacteria that then seeds the shunt. Community-acquired bacterial meningitis cases have been observed in patients with VP shunts and should also be considered.

5.2.4 Microbiology

The overwhelming majority of shunt infections are bacterial and caused by gram-positive organisms that comprise normal skin flora, with coagulase-negative *Staphylococcus* (CONS) bacteria accounting for 60–70% of cases [8]. *Staphylococcus aureus* represents an additional 20–30% of infected VP shunts. Infections by gram-negative organisms are more commonly seen in late-onset infections, with distal catheter infections caused by abdominal peritonitis or bowel perforation. Slow-growing organisms such as *Cutibacterium acnes* (previously known as *Propionibacterium acnes*) and *Corynebacterium* can be seen in indolent infections and are another important category of organisms to consider [9].

5.2.5 Signs and Symptoms

The clinical manifestations of VP shunt infections may range depending on the organism involved and how the infection occurred. As a general principle, none of the following clinical symptoms in isolation are sufficiently sensitive nor specific and should not be utilized independently to determine the likelihood of an infection.

Some patients may present with typical findings associated with bacterial meningitis including classic signs of meningismus (e.g., neck stiffness, bulging fontanelle, cranial nerve palsies) or with more subtle clues that may be confused with other more common diagnoses (such as viral infections or even gastroenteritis). Fever (particularly in the absence of another clear source), progressive headache, nausea, vomiting, lethargy, and altered mental status should clue the provider to consider a shunt infection, particularly in those with recent shunt placement as discussed above. Abdominal tenderness and pain may represent distal catheter infections and should prompt an evaluation for peritonitis from bowel perforation or, in rare instances, infected abdominal pseudocysts. Erythema, tenderness, and edema of the skin overlying a shunt tract are also significant causes for concern.

As some shunt infections are caused by slow-growing organisms that cause a limited inflammatory response, some patients present with only malaise or low-grade intermittent fevers. The classic findings of meningitis are not always present in infections with these organisms, and significant overlap with the more subtle and subacute findings seen in shunt malfunctions may be seen. Notably, shunt infection is an important risk factor for shunt malfunction, and the two diagnoses are often noted to coexist.

5.2.6 Workup and Diagnosis

Evaluation of the CSF via percutaneous needle aspiration of shunt fluid should be conducted by an experienced neurosurgeon, as the procedure involves a risk for causing infection. In cases of relatively low suspicion for shunt infection, lumbar puncture is a preferable method for CSF evaluation as part of the workup and can be performed by any physician trained in this procedure.

Culture of CSF from a shunt is considered to be the gold-standard and most definitive method to diagnose a VP shunt infection and should be performed as a component of the infectious workup. CSF gram stain, cell counts, glucose, and protein should also be ordered. In isolation, none of the CSF parameters outside of the bacterial culture are sufficiently sensitive or specific to be reliable indicators to rule infections in or out; however, they may offer clues as to the likelihood of an infected shunt. Importantly, normal CSF studies do not necessarily exclude the possibility of CSF shunt infection.

CSF samples should be obtained prior to the administration of antibiotics outside of the setting of severe sepsis, as the utility of CSF culture decreases in pre-treated samples.

Additional diagnostic workup may include gadolinium-enhanced and diffusion-weighted MRI, which can reveal findings associated with meningitis, abscess, or ventriculitis. Since infected shunts typically require removal, stereotactic protocol imaging may also be useful for operative planning. For those patients with abdominal symptoms or findings on physical exam, ultrasound or CT scans of the abdomen should be obtained.

5.2.7 Management

Initial management of VP shunt infections involves the administration of systemic antibiotics at meningitic dosing for empiric treatment until culture results are available to guide the tailoring of antibiotic choice. Owing to the high rates of gram-positive infections and the increasing incidence of methicillin-resistant staphylococci (MRSA), vancomycin is an appropriate choice as an initial antibiotic, in combination with a beta-lactam with gram-negative and pseudomonal coverage (typically cefepime, ceftazidime, or meropenem is recommended) [7]. Narrowing of antibiotics should be done as soon as culture-confirmed organisms and sensitivities are known.

Definitive management of infected VP shunts should include consultation with a neurosurgeon and infectious disease specialist. Management most commonly involves a combination of systemic antibiotic therapy and removal of all components of the infected shunt with placement of a temporary external ventricular drain. In general, management of a CSF shunt infection without shunt hardware removal is strongly discouraged given high failure rates seen with this approach. Decisions regarding the duration of antibiotics and timing of shunt replacement may vary as they take into consideration the organism involved, severity and extent of the infection, CSF infection clearance, as well as other individualized patient-specific factors.

5.3 *Other Complications*

Intracranial hemorrhage and neurologic injury can be seen in the immediate postoperative period after shunt insertion.

Wound dehiscence and CSF leakage are another subset of early postoperative complications. Both findings are taken to represent VP shunt infection and are most commonly treated as such.

Abdominal organ perforation (stomach, small/large bowel, bladder, or uterus) can occur during surgery or, rarely, with delayed presentation from persistent contact causing erosion of the tubing into visceral organs. Abdominal pseudocyst formation is another rare but notable intra-abdominal complication. Accumulation of CSF in the peritoneum can lead to the development of a cyst-like structure, which can then lead to either obstructive symptoms or infection of the shunt series. This finding is typically seen on shunt series X-rays, and, if identified, they are further evaluated with ultrasound.

6 Review Questions

1. A 15-month-old baby boy is brought in by parents to the emergency department with a chief complaint of irritability and poor feeding. His parents deny recording any fevers. He was born full term with congenital hydrocephalus, and a VP shunt was placed shortly after birth. On exam, he has normal vital signs for age. He appears sleepy but awakens to exam and moves all extremities symmetrically. There is no overlying swelling or erythema along his shunt catheter. Which of the following should be included as a part of his workup?

   (A) CSF culture
   (B) Rapid-sequence MRI of the brain
   (C) X-ray shunt series
   (D) Both B and C
   (E) A, B, and C

2. A 16-year-old girl born at 27 weeks gestational age with intraventricular hemorrhage of prematurity complicated by posthemorrhagic hydrocephalus status post

VP shunt (most recently revised 2 years ago), epilepsy, intellectual disability, chronic constipation, and recurrent urinary tract infections presents to the emergency department with a 1-day history of vomiting and increased seizure frequency from baseline. The differential diagnosis includes all of the following, except:

(A) Shunt infection
(B) Shunt malfunction
(C) Urinary tract infection
(D) Abdominal pseudocyst
(E) Viral syndrome

7 Answers

1. **D**. Rapid-sequence MRI of the brain and X-ray shunt series. Shunt malfunction can occur as both an early and late complication and should be evaluated via MRI brain and X-rays of the shunt catheter. Shunt infections most commonly occur within the first 6 months after placement and would be less likely in this case.
2. **D**. Abdominal pseudocyst. Abdominal pseudocyst usually does not present with fever unless it is secondarily infected, which is very rare.

8 Takeaway Points

1. Common ventricular shunt complications include shunt malfunction and shunt infections.
2. Presentation of shunt malfunction generally involves symptoms of increased intracranial pressure, though these can be nonspecific in infants and younger children.
3. Imaging workup for suspected shunt malfunction includes rapid-sequence MRI and X-ray shunt series.
4. CSF, as part of the infectious workup, can be obtained through a shunt tap in cases of high suspicion for shunt infection.
5. Management of shunt malfunction requires urgent neurosurgical intervention for the management of intracranial hypertension.
6. Management of shunt infections requires a combination of systemic broad-spectrum antibiotics and removal of the infected hardware for definitive management.

References

1. Frassanito P, Tamburrini G, Di Rocco C. Surgical treatment of hydrocephalus based on CSF shunt devices. In: Di Rocco C. Pang D, Rutka J. (eds) Textbook of Pediatric Neurosurgery. Springer. Cham. 2020. https://doi.org/10.1007/978-3-319-72168-2_25.
2. Aschoff A. In-Depth View: Functional characteristics of CSF shunt devices (Pros and Cons). In: Di Rocco C, Pang D, Rutka J. (eds) Textbook of Pediatric Neurosurgery. Springer. Cham. 2020. https://doi.org/10.1007/978-3-319-72168-2_26.
3. Mottolese C, Beuriat PA, Szathmari A, Di Rocco F. Complications related to the treatment of hydrocephalus with extrathecal cerebrospinal fluid shunts. In: Di Rocco C, Pang D, Rutka J. (eds) Textbook of Pediatric Neurosurgery. 2020. Springer. Cham. https://doi.org/10.1007/978-3-319-72168-2_33.
4. Kalra R, Kestle J. Congenital and developmental cerebral disorders: 10. Treatment of hydrocephalus with shunts. In: Albright L, Pollack I, Adelson D. (eds) Principles and practice of pediatric neurosurgery. 3rd ed. Stuttgart: Georg Thieme Verlag. 2015. https://doi.org/10.1055/b-0034-98050.
5. Frassanito P, Peraio S, Di Rocco C. Late complications of shunts. In: Di Rocco C, Pang D, Rutka J. (eds) Textbook of Pediatric Neurosurgery. Springer. Cham. 2020. https://doi.org/10.1007/978-3-319-72168-2_34.
6. Thompson D, Hartley J. Shunt infections. In: Albright L, Pollack I, Adelson D. (eds) Principles and practice of pediatric neurosurgery. 3rd ed. Stuttgart: Georg Thieme Verlag. 2015. https://doi.org/10.1055/b-0034-98117.
7. Tunkel AR, et al. 2017 infectious diseases society of America's clinical practice guidelines for healthcare-associated ventriculitis and meningitis. Clin Infect Dis. 2017;64(6):e34–65. https://doi.org/10.1093/cid/ciw861.
8. Cherry J, Demmler-Harrison GJ, Kaplan SL, Steinbach WJ, Hotez P. Feigin and Cherry's textbook of pediatric infectious diseases. 8th ed. Amsterdam: Elsevier – OHCE; 2018. https://bookshelf.health.elsevier.com/books/9780323392822
9. Long SS, et al. Principles and practice of pediatric infectious diseases E-book. 6th ed. Available from: Elsevier eBooks+. Elsevier – OHCE, 2022.

An Adolescent with an Ostomy and Abdominal Pain

Marie Dawlett and Amy Gonzalez

1 Case

A 17-year-old male recently diagnosed with ulcerative colitis (UC) presents to the emergency department for abdominal pain and nausea. His UC has been refractory to medical management (steroids and biologic agents). He underwent proctocolectomy with ileal pouch-anal anastomosis (IPAA) and temporary loop ileostomy 4 months ago due to his refractory disease course. Last night, he developed severe abdominal pain and nausea with significantly reduced output into his ileostomy bag. He has not been able to eat or drink in over 12 h. He is afebrile with a heart rate of 135, a respiratory rate of 20, and a blood pressure of 140/85. On exam, he is thin and pale with a distended abdomen that is diffusely tender to palpation with guarding and hyperactive bowel sounds. He has a slightly delayed capillary refill of 3 s. On inspection of the ileostomy site, there is a moderate-sized bulge surrounding the ostomy site. His physical examination is otherwise unremarkable. Abdominal radiography is obtained and demonstrates diffuse dilated loops of small bowel, measuring up to 5 cm in diameter. IV access is initiated, a normal saline bolus is given, and the surgery team is notified.

2 Discussion Questions

1. What is the most likely diagnosis for this patient?
2. What is the next best step in the management?
3. What are the potential complications in a patient with an ostomy?

M. Dawlett (✉) · A. Gonzalez
Department of Pediatrics, University of Texas Medical Branch, Galveston, TX, USA
e-mail: mfdawlet@utmb.edu; algonzal@utmb.edu

A. Kamzan et al. (eds.), *Children with Medical Complexity in the Emergency Department*, https://doi.org/10.1007/978-3-031-62517-6_17

3 Case Answers

1. The most likely diagnosis for this patient is a small bowel obstruction secondary to an incarcerated parastomal herniation. The severe pain, decreased output from the ileostomy, dilated bowel loops on imaging, and physical examination of the stoma (describing the bulge at the ostomy site) all support this diagnosis.
2. The next best step in the management of this patient is surgical correction of the obstruction.
3. The potential complications in a patient with an ostomy include stomal stenosis, peristomal skin complications such as infection, stomal retraction, stomal prolapse, peristomal hernia, bleeding at the site of the stoma, and dehydration from high-output fluid loss.

4 Learning Objectives

1. Describe the types of intestinal ostomies.
2. Outline ostomy-related complications, in relation to the timing of ostomy creation and type of ostomy.

5 Discussion

The patient in the vignette underwent total proctocolectomy (TPC) with ileal pouch-anal anastomosis (IPAA), which is an effective treatment for patients with ulcerative colitis (UC) refractory to medical management. He is presenting with signs and symptoms of an intestinal obstruction, most likely secondary to an incarcerated parastomal hernia.

An ostomy is a surgical procedure that creates an opening, called a stoma, on the abdomen to divert the colon (colostomy) or the small intestine, specifically the ileum (ileostomy), through the abdominal wall. It is performed when a portion of the colon or rectum needs to be bypassed or removed in the management of a variety of pathologic conditions including inflammatory bowel diseases, gastrointestinal malignancies, bowel obstructions, perforations, and trauma. The type of stoma, location of the stoma, and timing of the stoma creation determine the complication profile and the subsequent management.

The stoma allows waste products to exit the body and be collected in an external bag or pouch instead of passing through the rectum and anus. Colostomies and ileostomies can be temporary or permanent, and they provide a means for individuals to manage their bowel movements and maintain their quality of life. However, as with all ostomies, complications may arise, and providers should be able to identify these complications. The reported incidence of stomal complications ranges from 21% to 70%.

There are several different types of colostomies, which are named based on the location of the stoma and the portion of the colon involved.

In an ascending colostomy or transverse colostomy, the stoma is created from the ascending colon and the transverse colon, respectively. An ascending colostomy is a rare type of colostomy that will produce liquid stool that contains many digestive enzymes, and the peristomal skin must be protected from the stool at all times. Output from a transverse colostomy is typically more formed but still soft as it contains a lot of water because it has not yet traveled through much of the colon.

There are two main types of transverse colostomies including loop colostomy and double-barrel colostomy. In a loop colostomy, a loop of the transverse colon is brought out through the abdominal wall and will create what looks like a large stoma, but actually has two openings: one functioning stoma and the other nonfunctioning or diverted. The functioning stoma allows waste to pass through, while the nonfunctioning stoma is typically closed or diverted temporarily and may produce mucus. In a double-barrel colostomy, the transverse colon is divided into two separate stomas that may or may not be separated by skin. Waste is expelled through the proximal stoma, and the separate distal stoma is either closed or diverted and may produce mucus (called a mucous fistula).

Finally, there is a descending or sigmoid colostomy in which the stoma is created from the descending or sigmoid colon. This is the most common type of colostomy, and because there is more working colon, the stool output is firm and often on a more regular schedule.

Loop ileostomies and end ileostomies are the two most common types of standard ileostomies. Ileostomies are often present in the right abdomen and are smaller in size, producing loose, liquid stool. The choice between loop and end ileostomy depends on various factors, including the specific medical condition, the anticipated duration of the ileostomy, and the overall health of the patient.

In a loop ileostomy, a loop of the small intestine, usually the ileum, is brought to the surface of the abdomen and then divided creating two openings, one functioning stoma and the other temporarily closed. Loop ileostomies are often temporary and may be used to divert stool away from a diseased or healing portion of the intestine.

In contrast, in an end ileostomy, the ileum is completely divided, and the open end is brought out directly to the surface of the abdomen as the stoma. End ileostomies are more often permanent and are typically created when the entire colon or rectum is removed or nonfunctional.

End ileostomies and end colostomies are associated with lower complication rates than loop ostomies. Complications also differ depending on whether they occur in the immediate postoperative period, early (less than 3 months postoperatively) or late (greater than 3 months postoperatively) (Table 1).

The most common early complications of stoma creation include high-output fluid loss, improper stoma site selection, vascular compromise/stomal ischemia/necrosis, retraction, peristomal skin irritation, peristomal infection/abscess/fistula, acute parastomal herniation, and early postoperative bowel obstruction. Late complications (>3 months) include parastomal herniation, stoma prolapse, and stomal stenosis.

Table 1 Ostomy complications

Immediately post-op	Early (<3 months)	Late (>3 months)
• Bowel obstruction	• Fluid loss, electrolyte derangement • Improper site selection • Stomal ischemia/necrosis • Retraction • Peristomal skin irritation • Infection/abscess/fistula • Bowel obstruction	• Peristomal herniation • Stoma prolapse • Stomal stenosis

Peristomal skin problems are common and can occur at any time from a variety of causes including chemical injury from leakage of stoma effluent, mucocutaneous separation, irritation from adhesive stripping from repeated appliance application, contact dermatitis, infection, or pyoderma gangrenosum.

Stomal retraction is a complication commonly defined as a stoma that terminates >0.5 cm below the skin surface within 6 weeks of formation most frequently caused by tension on the bowel or its mesentery. It can also be caused by poor wound healing seen in patients that are malnourished, obese, or on corticosteroids. Stomal retraction can often lead to additional complications including leakage and peristomal skin irritation, mucocutaneous separation, and peristomal abscess.

Stomal necrosis due to vascular compromise ranges from mild ischemia to infarction and intestinal necrosis due to ligation of arterial supply or inadequate collateral arterial circulation. Necrosis may also arise from venous outflow obstruction leading to significant venous congestion and compromised bowel perfusion. If the mucosa appears dark or grayish, it should be considered compromised. When assessing the vascular integrity of a stoma, transillumination with a flashlight can demonstrate viability. The flashlight is placed in direct contact with the stoma, and the viable stoma will transilluminate red, while failure to transilluminate generally indicates that the stoma requires revision. Clinical signs include pain around the stoma, abdominal pain, fever, and signs of peritonitis.

Stomal stenosis is most commonly seen with end colostomies and often occurs due to bowel edema, small trephine size, early mucocutaneous separation, and retraction. Mild stenosis can be managed with decompression with large-bore rubber catheters; however, local revision with creation of a new tension-free stoma is needed with more severe stenoses.

A **parastomal hernia** is also most commonly seen with end colostomies and is defined as an incisional hernia that develops through the abdominal wall defect at the stoma site. An acute parastomal herniation can lead to intestinal obstruction, and when it occurs in the immediate postoperative period, it is usually caused by the creation of a too large facial defect. Clinical signs include nausea and emesis associated with a lump or mass adjacent to the stoma. Other clinical findings seen with a bowel obstruction include fever, leukocytosis, and presence of air-fluid levels on an upright abdominal radiograph. Management of a parastomal herniation causing bowel obstruction requires urgent reoperation with reduction of the hernia, resection of nonviable bowel if applicable, and revision of the fascial opening.

Parastomal infection of a mature stoma site usually results from local folliculitis or potentially from recurrent inflammatory bowel disease. Peristomal abscesses generally require that the abscess cavity be drained. After drainage, the patient is at higher risk for fistula formation.

Finally, one of the most common early complications is **high-output fluid loss**, which can lead to dehydration. Total volume of output fluid more than 1.5–2 L/day for adolescents and more than 20–30 ml/kg/day for infants and children is considered high output. These patients can present with electrolyte abnormalities including hypokalemia, non-anion gap metabolic acidosis, and hyponatremia and can have subsequent symptoms of confusion and lethargy. Fluid resuscitation and electrolyte management are key to management along with pharmacologic treatment aimed at decreasing motility as necessary. Avoiding meals high in fat and simple sugar content and increasing fiber intake to increase the thickness of the ileostomy effluent can also be recommended.

6 Review Questions

1. A 17-year-old patient with cerebral palsy and global intestinal dysmotility has an end colostomy in place due to recurrent episodes of fecal impaction. He presents with a 2-day history of fever, pain at the stomal site, guarding, and abdominal distention. On inspection of the intestinal mucosa, it does not transilluminate, and the mucosa appears dark. What is the most likely diagnosis?

   (A) Parastomal infection
   (B) Stomal necrosis
   (C) Stomal retraction
   (D) Stomal stenosis

2. In what type of colostomy would you expect that the stool output is mostly liquid?

   (A) Ascending colostomy
   (B) Descending colostomy
   (C) Transverse colostomy
   (D) Sigmoid colostomy

3. A 13-year-old patient with a loop ileostomy created 2 weeks ago presents to the ED with lethargy, confusion, tachycardia, and decreased urine output. He has had a significant increase in ostomy output, but his family has not measured quantity. What is the most likely electrolyte abnormality you would expect to see when labs are ordered?

   (A) Hyponatremia
   (B) Hyperglycemia
   (C) Hyperkalemia
   (D) Hyperphosphatemia

7 Answers

1. **B**. This patient is presenting with stomal necrosis. He has peritoneal signs and dark appearance of the mucosa that does not transilluminate. While parastomal infection can also cause fever, the mucosa is typically viable and will transilluminate. Stomal retraction is identified by observing the stoma >0.5 cm below the skin surface, and stomal stenosis will be identifiable based on the small aperture of the stoma.
2. **A.** An ascending colostomy would be expected to have mostly liquid stools, because the majority of water absorption has not yet occurred. In ostomies that are more distal, the stool output will contain less water and thus be more solid.
3. **A.** You can expect to see hyponatremia, hypophosphatemia, and hypokalemia in a patient with a high-output ostomy. These patients will often require hospitalization for fluid resuscitation and electrolyte replacement.

8 Takeaway Points

1. A parastomal hernia should be considered as a cause of small bowel obstruction in any patient with an ostomy.
2. Consider parastomal infection or parastomal hernia with obstruction when patients with stomas present with fever.
3. High-output ostomies (>1.5–2 L/day for adolescents and >20–30 ml/kg for infants/children) can cause severe dehydration and electrolyte abnormalities.

Further Reading

Kann BR. Early stomal complications. Clin Colon Rectal Surg. 2008;21(1):23–30. https://doi.org/10.1055/s-2008-1055318.

Murken DR, Bleier JIS. Ostomy-related complications. Clin Colon Rectal Surg. 2019;32(3):176–82. https://doi.org/10.1055/s-0038-1676995. Epub 2019 Apr 2.

A Patient with a Heart Transplant and Abdominal Pain

Helen Zhou, Majid Husain, and Juan Alejos

1 Case

An 8-year-old female with a history of dilated cardiomyopathy status post orthotopic heart transplant with an ABO-compatible heart at 2 years of age presents to the emergency room with 3 days of general malaise. She also reports abdominal pain and a dry cough. She does not have fever, rhinorrhea, nausea, vomiting, or diarrhea. She denies any chest pain, shortness of breath, or palpitations. She has had no sick contacts or recent travel.

Her last echocardiogram and cardiac catheterization 4 months prior revealed normal biventricular function and normal hemodynamics without any evidence of coronary artery vasculopathy, respectively. Her endomyocardial biopsy at that time was negative for cellular and antibody-mediated rejection. She has been relatively stable for the past few months although her tacrolimus trough level has not been at goal at the last clinic visit secondary to an episode of viral gastroenteritis 1 week ago. She has been compliant with her posttransplant medications, including antihypertensives, immunosuppressants, and immunoprophylaxis.

On her initial examination, she is afebrile, tachycardic to 120 beats/min, with a normal blood pressure and oxygen saturation level. She appears fatigued and has a prominent S3 with a laterally displaced point of maximum impulse (PMI). Her respiratory exam shows crackles bilaterally in her lung bases and mildly increased work of breathing. Her abdominal exam reveals a tender right upper quadrant with hepatomegaly extending 4 cm below the costal margin. Her extremities are warm but with diminished pulses and prolonged capillary refill. There is no significant edema. Her neurologic examination and mental status are at baseline.

H. Zhou (✉) · M. Husain · J. Alejos
Department of Pediatrics, UCLA Mattel Children's Hospital, Los Angeles, CA, USA
e-mail: helenzhou@mednet.ucla.edu; majidhusain@mednet.ucla.edu; jalejos@mednet.ucla.edu

A. Kamzan et al. (eds.), *Children with Medical Complexity in the Emergency Department*, https://doi.org/10.1007/978-3-031-62517-6_18

2 Discussion Questions

1. What is on the differential diagnosis?
2. How does cardiac transplant rejection present?
3. What is the initial workup for cardiac rejection?

3 Case Answers

1. The differential for this patient is very broad including, but not limited to, acute infectious processes, appendicitis, gallstones, tacrolimus toxicity, but most importantly acute cardiac rejection.
2. Cardiac rejection can present with symptoms ranging from mild and nonspecific to severe shock and heart failure.
3. The initial workup for rejection includes a thorough history, exam, labs including brain natriuretic peptide (BNP) and troponin, electrocardiogram (EKG), and echocardiogram. Expert consultation with pediatric transplant cardiology should be part of the initial conversation to determine if additional workup is indicated.

4 Learning Objectives

1. Understand the differential for general malaise in children with heart transplants
2. Describe the initial presentation of heart transplant rejection
3. Understand initial workup of rejection in the ED

5 Discussion

5.1 *Background*

Pediatric heart transplant is the ultimate option in the treatment of end-stage heart disease refractory to maximum medical therapy or surgical management. Pediatric heart transplants currently comprise approximately 10% of total cases of heart transplantation [1]. The primary diagnosis and indications vary by age. In infants younger than 1 year of age, both unrepaired and palliated complex congenital heart disease (CHD) is the most common underlying diagnosis, specifically single-ventricle pathology such as hypoplastic left heart syndrome (HLHS) [2]. Despite advances in surgical techniques and improved postsurgical outcomes in CHD, transplantation remains an important option for those patients with failed palliation or significant ventricular dysfunction. Cardiomyopathy (CMY), specifically dilated cardiomyopathy (DCM), is the most common indication for transplantation in older children [2]. Overall, cardiomyopathy (dilated, hypertrophic, or restrictive) collectively remains the most common indication for pediatric heart transplantation.

Posttransplantation, the highest risk of death, is during the first year. Those that survived had a median survival of over 15 years across all age groups. The most recent data from the International Society for Heart and Lung Transplantation (ISHLT) demonstrates a median survival of approximately 22 years in patients <1 year of age at transplantation, 18 years for those aged 1–5, 14 years for those 6–10 years, and 13 years for adolescents [3, 4]. While survival posttransplantation is improving, graft failure, rejection, infection, and cardiac allograft vasculopathy are major causes of death or need for re-transplantation [5]. Not surprisingly, this vulnerable population requires close monitoring and careful evaluation when presenting to the emergency department with a wide array of symptoms.

In this chapter, we will specifically focus on rejection. We will briefly review its pathophysiology, presenting symptoms, initial management, and overall management plan.

5.2 *Heart Transplant Rejection*

5.2.1 Pathophysiology and Timing

Transplant rejection is an immune-mediated phenomenon and a direct result of the complex interactions between donor antigens and the recipient immune system's response. Despite careful selection and matching of the donor to the recipient, posttransplant induction therapy, and maintenance immunotherapy, rejection remains an ongoing concern [3–6]. It can occur as early as intra/perioperatively (hyperacute), in weeks to several months posttransplant (acute), or several months to years posttransplantation (chronic) [7]. While most episodes of rejection occur within the first 3 months after transplantation [8], it is important to note that rejection can occur at any time posttransplantation. Hyperacute rejection is related to blood group incompatibility (ABO incompatibility) or preformed antibodies in the recipient against donor antigens [7]. As expected, this form of rejection is not seen in the ED as it occurs during intraoperative or in the immediate postoperative period. Acute rejection can occur via a cellular (cytotoxic T-cells) or humoral (antibody-mediated) mechanism. Chronic rejection is related to helper T-cells and plasma cells [7]. Collectively, the recipient response to donor antigens results in a significant inflammatory response with consequent endothelial, vascular, and myocardial damage.

The specific immunochemical interactions between human leukocyte antigens (HLAs), genes in major histocompatibility complexes (MHCs) that help code for proteins that differentiate between self and non-self, and innate and adaptive immune system of the recipient that lead to the various types of rejection are beyond the scope of this chapter [9].

Risk factors for hyperacute rejection are mitigated by careful selection as mentioned above and are extremely rare in the modern era. Risk factors for acute and chronic rejection included non-white race, older recipient age, early rejection with hemodynamic compromise, recipient without congenital heart disease, and male donor [1, 3, 5, 6, 10].

The transplant team performs routine rejection surveillance via outpatient clinic visits, serial echocardiograms, and right-heart catheterization with endomyocardial biopsy (EMB) at pre-planned intervals. In addition to EMB, assays to monitor donor-derived cell-free DNA via peripheral blood sampling may also be done [11].

5.2.2 Presentation

Clinical Presentation

Heart transplant rejection in patients can present with a variety of symptoms and at any time during their posttransplant course [12, 13]. These symptoms are often vague and nonspecific, making the diagnosis of rejection challenging. Therefore, it is imperative to maintain a high index of suspicion and perform a thorough evaluation when assessing these unique patients.

The symptoms can range from mild to severe as highlighted in Table 1. Notably, the symptoms also vary by age. For example, an infant with rejection may present with feeding intolerance and irritability. Adolescent patients by comparison may simply report not feeling well; nausea and vomiting are commonly reported symptoms. Regardless of age, a complete review of systems is indicated to elucidate clues of rejection. Consultation with the pediatric transplant cardiologist is imperative for any patient presenting to the ED regardless of the chief complaint because oftentimes the transplant team can provide additional perspective and is aware of the patient's clinical course and its subtleties.

Notably, headache, irritability, and head/neck venous distention may be related to SVC obstruction due to thrombosis or narrowing of surgical anastomosis. The risk is increased in patients with bicaval anastomosis during transplant or with a history of Glenn/bidirectional cavopulmonary anastomosis.

Table 1 Clinical symptoms of cardiac rejection

Mild	Moderate	Severe
Asymptomatic	Decreased appetite/PO intake	Chest pain
Malaise	Fatigue/lethargy	Dyspnea
Overall not feeling well	Nausea/vomiting	Shock
	Abdominal pain/fullness	Changes in mental status
	Fever/flu-like symptoms	
	Weight gain/edema	
	Decreased urine output	
	Decreased exercise tolerance	
	Palpitations	

Differential Diagnosis

Given the vague and nonspecific symptoms of transplant rejection, the differential remains very broad and includes common pediatric diseases as well as cardiac transplant-specific diagnoses. Below we will discuss the cardiac transplant-specific diagnoses.

Children with heart transplants are at increased risk for infections secondary to their immunosuppressive therapies, history of major surgical procedures, potential for prosthetic material or devices, and abnormal pulmonary and cardiac function from underlying cardiac disease (congenital heart disease) [3, 12, 13]. They are at risk for serious bacterial infections like *Streptococcus pneumoniae* and *Staphylococcus aureus*, viral infections especially Epstein-Barr virus (EBV) and cytomegalovirus (CMV), fungal infections, and opportunistic infections like *Pneumocystis jirovecii* pneumonia (PCP) [3].

Tacrolimus toxicity can present with neurologic symptoms of tremulousness, headache, irritability, altered consciousness, visual disturbances, and seizures [14]. These symptoms can occur in isolation or in concert with each other. Tacrolimus is a calcineurin inhibitor that is one of the most commonly used immunosuppressive therapies. It is monitored with a trough serum level that is typically drawn 30 min prior to the medication being administered. Goal levels are unique to each patient, and patients can show signs of toxicity at any level. Other typical findings with tacrolimus toxicity are headache, acute kidney injury, hypertension, hypomagnesemia, hyperkalemia, hyperglycemia, thrombocytopenia, and leukopenia [14]. Tacrolimus absorption and metabolism are also affected by many medications. Antifungals (i.e., fluconazole), macrolides, metoclopramide, amiodarone, and calcium channel blockers may increase serum tacrolimus levels, while antiepileptics (phenytoin, phenobarbital, carbamazepine) and antibiotics (trimethoprim/sulfamethoxazole, nafcillin) may decrease serum levels. Tacrolimus levels can also increase when a patient has an acute infection or diarrhea. Levels are increased with certain foods like grapefruit and pomegranate or prolonged fasting. While elevated tacrolimus levels can cause signs of toxicity, low serum levels increase the risk of rejection. Among transplanted patients, adolescents are at high risk for medication nonadherence resulting in low serum levels and consequent signs and symptoms of rejection. Conversely, supratherapeutic levels of the drug result in neurotoxicity in the form of posterior reversible encephalopathy syndrome (PRES). Other common immunosuppressants used include sirolimus, which can cause mouth sores and diarrhea, and mycophenolate, which can cause significant gastrointestinal symptoms and leukopenia [14].

Notably, posttransplant lymphoproliferative disease (PTLD) should be highest on the differential for a transplanted patient presenting with B-symptoms of fever, generalized malaise, night sweats, and weight loss. PTLD is a major cause of morbidity and mortality in pediatric heart transplant recipients. It affects approximately 10% of the surviving patients 10 years after transplantation and results in graft rejection and ultimately graft loss due to having to reduce immunosuppression to treat the PTLD [15, 16].

5.2.3 Initial Workup and Management

The initial workup starts with obtaining a thorough history and physical examination. All patients and/or their caregivers should have a "passport" outlining the specifics regarding their heart transplantation and current care. This may be linked to the electronic health record if the patient received their transplant at the same institution. Referencing this document allows providers to quickly gain insight into the patient's history, especially as it pertains to timing since transplantation and previous episodes of rejection. Triaging based on this is a prudent approach to care for these complex patients.

Given the wide range of presentation, the patient may appear well with an otherwise reassuring or unremarkable physical exam. Those with moderate to severe symptoms will naturally appear unwell. Vital signs may show tachycardia or hypertension. On physical exam, the patient may have a new gallop heard on the cardiac auscultation. There may also be signs of acute heart failure including but not limited to jugular venous distention (JVD), hepatomegaly, or pulmonary crackles related to pulmonary edema.

Initial workup includes EKG, echocardiogram, chest X-ray, and blood work including BNP (or NT proBNP based on institutional preference), troponin, complete blood count, renal/liver function, electrolytes, and immunosuppression medication levels such as tacrolimus and sirolimus if timing is appropriate (e.g., trough level). Note that the immunosuppression levels may be difficult to interpret depending on the timing of lab draw relative to when the patient took the medication. Echocardiogram is considered to be the first-line complementary imaging tool in assessing rejection. However, the most definitive testing and current gold standard for rejection is endomyocardial biopsy—this will typically be reserved once the patient is thoroughly evaluated and its need is critically assessed. It is important to note that the severity of ventricular dysfunction may not correlate with the severity of rejection on endomyocardial biopsy or the patient's presenting symptoms (Table 2).

Table 2 Initial workup and correlated findings

Evaluation	Findings *(may occur in isolation or collectively)*
Physical exam	Tachycardia, new or worsening murmur, new gallop, signs of venous congestion (JVD, hepatomegaly, pulmonary crackles, edema)
Chest X-ray	Cardiomegaly and/or pulmonary edema, effusion
EKG	Low-voltage QRS signal. New arrhythmias. Note: Transplanted hearts are "denervated" and have a higher resting heart rate
Echocardiogram	Decreased ventricular function (systolic and diastolic), new pericardial effusion, worsening of mitral or tricuspid valve regurgitation, increased left ventricular wall thickness, myocardial echogenicity, reduced strain
Laboratory	Elevated BNP, sub/supratherapeutic immunosuppression levels, elevated blood urea nitrogen (BUN) or creatinine

Initial Management

After primary surveillance, immediately consult with the pediatric heart transplant cardiologist (locally or from the patient's transplant institution) for shared decision-making regardless of the initial presentation and severity of the symptoms. It is important to note that a transplanted heart varies anatomically and behaves physiologically different from a native heart. Therefore, interventions have to be calibrated accordingly.

The most likely intervention in a patient presenting with signs and symptoms of rejection but without hemodynamic compromise will be parenteral steroids [17] followed by the decision to admit to the pediatric ward versus the intensive care unit. Once the patient has been evaluated and stabilized appropriately in the ED, it would be prudent to transfer the patient to an institution equipped with a pediatric heart transplant team if needed.

Patients presenting with acute rejection with hemodynamic compromise will require judicious use of volume and inotropic support in addition to treatment for rejection. The treatment of rejection may consist of a pulse dose of steroids and a regimen consisting of anti-T-cell therapy, intravenous immunoglobulin, or rituximab [17]. Most of the immunotherapies will be administered once the patient is admitted. In general, avoid fluid boluses to reduce the risk of precipitating or worsening heart failure. If the heart function is normal by echocardiogram, consider small-volume boluses on a case-by-case basis.

6 Review Questions

1. A 13-month-old male with a history of hypoplastic left heart syndrome presents to the ED with increasing fussiness and tremors on post-op day 14 after an orthotopic heart transplant. His exam is at baseline. His immunosuppressants have been at goal. His labs show elevated BUN and creatinine, hypomagnesemia, hyperglycemia, and downtrending BNP. What most likely led to the development of his new symptoms?

   (A) Development of HLA antibodies
   (B) Starting fluconazole for a fungal infection
   (C) Acute kidney injury from over-diuresis
   (D) Subtherapeutic tacrolimus levels

2. A 16-year-old male with a history of a heart transplant as an infant presents with fever, cough, general malaise, chest pain, and dyspnea. Physical exam is significant for palpable lymph nodes. His echocardiogram showed normal left ventricular systolic function but impaired diastolic function. Which of the following is on his differential?

   (A) EBV viremia

(B) Posttransplant lymphoproliferative disorder
(C) Chronic heart rejection
(D) All of the above

3. A 9-year-old female with a history of dilated cardiomyopathy now status post orthotopic heart transplant 2 years prior presents to the emergency room with signs of new-onset heart failure with decreased exercise tolerance, pedal edema, and nausea. On exam, her temperature is 37.1 °C, heart rate is 124 beats/min, blood pressure is 110/74 mmHg, respiratory rate is 16 breaths/min, and oxygen saturation is 100% on room air. She has a new gallop and hepatomegaly concerning for heart rejection. What is the next best step in her workup and management?

   (A) Cardiac catheterization
   (B) Small bolus of fluids
   (C) Echocardiogram
   (D) Tacrolimus trough level

7 Answers

1. **B**. Starting fluconazole for a fungal infection. This patient is presenting with signs of tacrolimus toxicity likely related to starting fluconazole. Antifungals like fluconazole increase tacrolimus serum levels. Patients may show symptoms of toxicity at any level. Development of HLA antibodies leads to acute heart rejection, which can present with vague signs of fussiness but usually presents with increasing BNP and exam findings of tachycardia, new murmurs, or venous congestion. Acute kidney injury can lead to the electrolyte abnormalities like hypomagnesemia, hyper- or hypoglycemia, and elevated BUN and creatinine, but AKI is not likely to cause fussiness and tremors.
2. **D**. All of the above. The differential for general symptoms of fever, malaise, and dyspnea is very broad in a transplant patient. They are at risk for infections especially CMV and EBV due to immunosuppression. The highest risk for heart rejection is in the first 6 months to 2 years posttransplant; in fact, some studies suggest that the highest risk of transplant is within the first 3 months, though it can happen at any time in a patient's lifetime. PTLD often presents with nonspecific B symptoms like fevers, night sweats, and weight loss. On physical examination, you may find generalized lymphadenopathy. As it is a major cause of morbidity and mortality in solid-organ recipients, it is essential to have a high index of suspicion. All the answer options can present with general symptoms and signs of reduced heart function on echocardiogram. Further workup including lab studies and possibly endomyocardial biopsy is needed to further elucidate the cause.
3. **C**. Echocardiogram. The initial workup of heart transplant rejection in the ED should begin with an echocardiogram to compare her heart function to previous echocardiogram studies. While cardiac catheterization is the gold standard to

diagnose rejection, echocardiogram is the first-line imaging tool. This patient is stable with only tachycardia, so there is no need for emergent fluid resuscitation that could potentially worsen her heart function. While a tacrolimus trough level will be needed to determine if she had adequate level of immunosuppression, it would not diagnose her heart rejection. Rather, it may suggest rejection as a possible etiology of her symptoms if the appropriately timed trough levels are subtherapeutic.

8 Takeaway Points

1. Give parenteral methylprednisolone to a transplanted patient presenting to the ED with signs and symptoms of rejection. The benefits of prompt administration far outweigh the risks. Typical dose: 10 mg/kg IV daily ×3 days (max 500 mg/dose) followed by a taper.
2. Consultation with a pediatric transplant cardiologist is recommended for any patient presenting to the ED regardless of the chief complaint to ensure optimal care.
3. Primary evaluation of a pediatric patient post-orthotopic heart transplant presenting to the ED should include surveillance for heart transplant rejection, medication toxicity, and adherence with medication (especially in adolescent patients).
4. Evaluate for cardiac rejection in any pediatric patient post-orthotopic heart transplant that presents with symptoms that mimic common pediatric complaints (e.g., abdominal pain, vomiting, headache).
5. Clinical findings of acute/active rejection include:

    (a) Physical exam: New gallop (most sensitive), tachycardia, new or worsening murmurs of mitral or tricuspid valve regurgitation, or evidence of venous congestion (hepatomegaly, JVD, fine or coarse crackles on lung auscultation)
    (b) Chest X-ray: New or worsening cardiomegaly and/or pulmonary venous congestion
    (c) Echocardiography: Decreased ventricular function (systolic and diastolic), new pericardial effusion, worsening of mitral or tricuspid valve regurgitation, and increased wall thickness/mass
    (d) EKG: Low-voltage QRS signal (not diagnostic in isolation)
    (e) Laboratory: Elevated serum natriuretic peptide (BNP, NT-proBNP)

6. Headache, irritability, and head/neck venous distention may be related to SVC obstruction (thrombosis or narrowing of surgical anastomosis).
7. New-onset arrhythmia should raise suspicion for rejection (early posttransplant) or coronary artery vasculopathy (late posttransplant).

8. High serum levels of immunosuppressive drugs can cause:
   (a) Tacrolimus—seizures, irritability, tremulousness, AKI, hypomagnesemia
   (b) Sirolimus—diarrhea, mouth sores
   (c) Azathioprine/mycophenolate—GI symptoms (constipation, diarrhea, vomiting), leukopenia
9. Antifungals, macrolides, metoclopramide, amiodarone, and calcium channel blockers increase calcineurin inhibitor (tacrolimus, cyclosporin) serum levels. Certain antiepileptics (phenytoin, phenobarbital, carbamazepine) and antibiotics (trimethoprim-sulbactam, nafcillin) may decrease serum levels.
10. Nonspecific constitutional symptoms (malaise, weight loss, and fever of unknown origin) and physical exam findings of lymphadenopathy or an elevated EBV titer on laboratory evaluation should warrant evaluation of post-transplant lymphoproliferative disorder (PTLD).

References

1. Rossano JW, Dipchand AI, Edwards LB, Goldfarb S, Kucheryavaya AY, Levvey Rn BJ, Lund LH, Meiser B, Yusen RD, Stehlik J, International Society for Heart and Lung Transplantation. The Registry of the International Society for Heart and Lung Transplantation: nineteenth pediatric heart transplantation report-2016; Focus theme: primary diagnostic indications for transplant. J Heart Lung Transplant. 2016;35(10):1185–95. https://doi.org/10.1016/j.healun.2016.08.018. Epub 2016 Aug 21
2. Canter CE, Shaddy RE, Bernstein D, Hsu DT, Chrisant MR, Kirklin JK, Kanter KR, Higgins RS, Blume ED, Rosenthal DN, Boucek MM, Uzark KC, Friedman AH, Young JK, American Heart Association Council on Cardiovascular Disease in the Young; American Heart Association Council on Clinical Cardiology; American Heart Association Council on Cardiovascular Nursing; American Heart Association Council on Cardiovascular Surgery and Anesthesia; Quality of Care and Outcomes Research Interdisciplinary Working Group. Indications for heart transplantation in pediatric heart disease: a scientific statement from the American Heart Association Council on Cardiovascular Disease in the Young; the Councils on Clinical Cardiology, Cardiovascular Nursing, and Cardiovascular Surgery and Anesthesia; and the Quality of Care and Outcomes Research Interdisciplinary Working Group. Circulation. 2007;115(5):658–76. https://doi.org/10.1161/CIRCULATIONAHA.106.180449. Epub 2007 Jan 29. Erratum in: Circulation. 2007 Apr 3;115(13):e385. Friedman, Allen H [corrected to Friedman, Alan H].
3. Dipchand AI, Laks JA. Pediatric heart transplantation: long-term outcomes. Indian J Thorac Cardiovasc Surg. 2020;36(Suppl 2):175–89. https://doi.org/10.1007/s12055-019-00820-3. Epub 2019 May 29
4. Hayes D Jr, Cherikh WS, Chambers DC, Harhay MO, Khush KK, Lehman RR, Meiser B, Rossano JW, Hsich E, Potena L, Sadavarte A, Singh TP, Zuckermann A, Stehlik J, International Society for Heart and Lung Transplantation. The International Thoracic Organ Transplant Registry of the International Society for Heart and Lung Transplantation: twenty-second pediatric lung and heart-lung transplantation report-2019; Focus theme: donor and recipient size match. J Heart Lung Transplant. 2019;38(10):1015–27. https://doi.org/10.1016/j.healun.2019.08.003. Epub 2019 Aug 8.
5. Dipchand AI. Current state of pediatric cardiac transplantation. Ann Cardiothorac Surg. 2018;7(1):31–55. https://doi.org/10.21037/acs.2018.01.07.

6. Everitt MD, Pahl E, Schechtman KB, Zheng J, Ringewald JM, L'ecuyer T, Naftel DC, Kirklin JK, Blume ED, Bullock EA, Canter CE, Pediatric Heart Transplant Study Investigators. Rejection with hemodynamic compromise in the current era of pediatric heart transplantation: a multi-institutional study. J Heart Lung Transplant. 2011;30(3):282–8. https://doi.org/10.1016/j.healun.2010.08.031. Epub 2010 Oct 25
7. Moreau A, Varey E, Anegon I, Cuturi MC. Effector mechanisms of rejection. Cold Spring Harb Perspect Med. 2013;3(11):a015461. https://doi.org/10.1101/cshperspect.a015461.
8. Godown J, Cantor R, Koehl D, Cummings E, Vo JB, Dodd DA, Lytrivi I, Boyle GJ, Sutcliffe DL, Kleinmahon JA, Shih R, Urschel S, Das B, Carlo WF, Zuckerman WA, West SC, MA MC, Zinn MD, Simpson KE, Kindel SJ, Szmuszkovicz JR, Chrisant M, Auerbach SR, Carboni MP, Kirklin JK, Hsu DT. Practice variation in the diagnosis of acute rejection among pediatric heart transplant centers: an analysis of the pediatric heart transplant society (PHTS) registry. J Heart Lung Transplant. 2021;40(12):1550–9. https://doi.org/10.1016/j.healun.2021.08.002. Epub 2021 Aug 19
9. Ingulli E. Mechanism of cellular rejection in transplantation. Pediatr Nephrol. 2010;25(1):61–74. https://doi.org/10.1007/s00467-008-1020-x.
10. Chin C, Naftel DC, Singh TP, Blume ED, Luikart H, Bernstein D, Gamberg P, Kirklin JK, Morrow WR, Pediatric Heart Transplant Study Group. Risk factors for recurrent rejection in pediatric heart transplantation: a multicenter experience. J Heart Lung Transplant. 2004;23(2):178–85. https://doi.org/10.1016/S1053-2498(03)00059-7.
11. Feingold B, Rose-Felker K, West SC, Zinn MD, Berman P, Moninger A, Huston A, Stinner B, Xu Q, Zeevi A, Miller SA. Early findings after integration of donor-derived cell-free DNA into clinical care following pediatric heart transplantation. Pediatr Transplant. 2022;26(1):e14124. https://doi.org/10.1111/petr.14124. Epub 2021 Aug 22
12. Kirklin JK. Current challenges in pediatric heart transplantation for congenital heart disease. Curr Opin Organ Transplant. 2015;20(5):577–83. https://doi.org/10.1097/MOT.0000000000000238.
13. Thrush PT, Hoffman TM. Pediatric heart transplantation-indications and outcomes in the current era. J Thorac Dis. 2014;6(8):1080–96. https://doi.org/10.3978/j.issn.2072-1439.2014.06.16.
14. Khimji IA, Kazmerski TM, Webber SA. Immunosuppressive agents in pediatric heart transplantation. In: Munoz R, Schmitt CG, Roth SJ, da Cruz E, editors. Handbook of pediatric cardiovascular drugs. London: Springer; 2008. https://doi.org/10.1007/978-1-84628-953-8_8.
15. Chinnock R, Webber SA, Dipchand AI, Brown RN, George JF, Pediatric Heart Transplant Study. A 16-year multi-institutional study of the role of age and EBV status on PTLD incidence among pediatric heart transplant recipients. Am J Transplant. 2012;12(11):3061–8. https://doi.org/10.1111/j.1600-6143.2012.04197.x. Epub 2012 Oct 16
16. Abbas F, El Kossi M, Shaheen IS, Sharma A, Halawa A. Post-transplantation lymphoproliferative disorders: current concepts and future therapeutic approaches. World J Transplant. 2020;10(2):29–46. https://doi.org/10.5500/wjt.v10.i2.29.
17. Bansal N, Everitt MD, Nandi D, Spinner J, Conway J, Magnetta DA, Profita EL, Townsend M, Alejos JC, Deshpande SR. Clinical approach to acute cellular rejection from the pediatric heart transplant society. Pediatr Transplant. 2022;26(8):e14393. https://doi.org/10.1111/petr.14393.

Further Reading

Dipchand AI, Laks JA. Pediatric heart transplantation: long-term outcomes. Indian J Thorac Cardiovasc Surg. 2020;36(Suppl 2):175–89. https://doi.org/10.1007/s12055-019-00820-3. Epub 2019 May 29

International Society for Heart and Lung Transplantation (ISHLT) monograph series: volume 2 and 13—Pediatric heart transplantation (https://ishlt.org/publications-resources/publications/monograph-series).

Kirklin JK. Current challenges in pediatric heart transplantation for congenital heart disease. Curr Opin Organ Transplant. 2015;20(5):577–83. https://doi.org/10.1097/MOT.0000000000000238.

Rossano JW, Dipchand AI, Edwards LB, Goldfarb S, Kucheryavaya AY, Levvey Rn BJ, Lund LH, Meiser B, Yusen RD, Stehlik J, International Society for Heart and Lung Transplantation. The Registry of the International Society for Heart and Lung Transplantation: nineteenth pediatric heart transplantation report-2016; Focus theme: primary diagnostic indications for transplant. J Heart Lung Transplant. 2016;35(10):1185–95. https://doi.org/10.1016/j.healun.2016.08.018. Epub 2016 Aug 21.

A Renal Transplant Recipient with Elevated Blood Pressure and Loose Stool

Allison E. Williams and Elizabeth Spiwak

1 Case

An 8-year-old boy with a history of end-stage kidney disease secondary to posterior urethral valves status post living-related donor kidney transplant presents to his local community emergency department (ED) for diarrhea and hypertension. Three days ago, he began to have watery, but non-bloody diarrhea at home, approximately 5–6 episodes per day. He also reports some cramping abdominal pain intermittently but no vomiting. There is no fever. He has normal urine output and normal PO intake. Sick contacts include his sister who had mild diarrhea starting 2 days prior to his symptoms. Her symptoms resolved within 24 h. The patient was seen by his pediatrician where his blood pressure was noted to be 140/85. Due to symptoms and hypertension, he was sent to the ED. Past medical history includes kidney transplant 12 months ago. He is maintained on mycophenolate mofetil and tacrolimus for immunosuppression, with no missed doses of medication. There is no history of recent rejection episodes. There is no pertinent family history or social history, and no recent travel or reserve travel. Upon arrival to the ED, he is afebrile with a heart rate of 110 and a blood pressure of 135/80. His weight is 24 kg, which is 4% down from his last nephrology appointment 2 weeks prior. On exam, he is awake and alert, with no focal cardiac or pulmonary findings. Capillary refill is 2–3 s. His abdomen is soft, non-distended with initial reports of tenderness in all four quadrants. Surgical scar is well healed. There is no edema noted.

A. E. Williams (✉)
Department of Pediatrics, UPMC Children's Hospital of Pittsburgh, University of Pittsburgh School of Medicine, Pittsburgh, PA, USA
e-mail: allison.williams2@chp.edu

E. Spiwak
Department of Pediatrics, Peyton Manning Children's Hospital Indianapolis, Indianapolis, IN, USA
e-mail: elizabeth.spiwak@ascension.org

A. Kamzan et al. (eds.), *Children with Medical Complexity in the Emergency Department*, https://doi.org/10.1007/978-3-031-62517-6_19

2 Discussion Questions

1. What lab studies or imaging would you like for initial evaluation?
2. What is the next best step in management?
3. What complications of renal transplant should be anticipated in this patient?

3 Case Answers

1. Basic metabolic panel with magnesium and phosphorus levels, urinalysis with a urine culture. Consider obtaining stool cultures. While awaiting creatinine result, consider renal ultrasound.
2. Fluid resuscitation with 20 mL/kg of normal saline. Acetaminophen at 15 mg/kg for abdominal pain. Avoid nonsteroidal anti-inflammatory drugs (NSAIDs).
3. Complications that should be anticipated include immunosuppression medication side effect or toxicity, infection (including community-acquired infections such as viral vs. bacterial gastroenteritis, urinary tract infection, or pyelonephritis), and chronic rejection, though there is no history of rejection episodes.

4 Learning Objectives

1. Understand the complications of kidney transplantation.
2. Recognize abnormal signs and symptoms that may be present in patients with a history of kidney transplantation.
3. Understand initial management for stabilization of patients with a history of kidney transplantation.

5 Discussion

In the pediatric population, kidney transplantation is the standard of care for children with end-stage renal disease (ESRD). Dialysis, either hemodialysis or peritoneal dialysis, is used as a bridge to transplantation. End-stage renal disease is caused by a wide variety of factors including congenital anomalies of the kidney and urinary tract, inherited genetic or metabolic disorders, and intrarenal acquired syndromes such as repeat infections, glomerulonephritis, and nephrotic syndrome among many others [1–3]. Ultimately, the benefits of improved quality of life and increased life expectancy with kidney transplantation outweigh the risks associated with the surgical procedure and posttransplant care. The most recent data from the Organ Procurement and Transplant Network in 2022 showed a total of over 700 pediatric kidney transplants performed. Of those transplants performed in patients younger than 18 years old, the majority were in children between the ages of 11 and 17 [4].

It is generally acceptable to divide complications of renal transplantation by timing posttransplant, such as the acute phase (first 30 days after transplantation), subacute phase (30–180 days after transplantation), and latent or chronic phase (after 180 days). Acute complications of kidney transplantation include bleeding, vessel injury, thrombosis, fistula, urinary leak/obstruction, wound complications, infections predominantly derived from the donor, and acute rejection. Acute complications will not be discussed in this chapter as they will most likely be treated by the tertiary care center where the transplantation occurred. Subacute and chronic infections are more commonly seen within the community hospitals. Subacute complications include infectious etiologies, but also rejection and recurrence of the original kidney disease. Chronic complications include the same etiologies as subacute complications with the addition of posttransplant lymphoproliferative disease. Infections are one of the most common complications experienced by kidney transplant recipients including bacterial, viral, fungal, and even parasitic etiologies. In addition to the increased risk of acquiring community infections, recipients are at risk for donor-derived infections and recurrence of primary latent infections such as herpes simplex virus or cytomegalovirus due to immunosuppressive therapy [1–3].

All patients who receive a solid-organ transplant must undergo induction and maintenance immunosuppression. There are exceptions to this rule, such as the recipient of a graft from a haplotype-identical living-related donor (i.e., identical twin) [5]; however, when evaluating patients with kidney transplantation, providers should assume that the patient is on immunosuppressive medication. Most maintenance immunosuppression therapies involve glucocorticoids (though some centers are steroid-sparing or steroid-free), an antiproliferative agent such as mycophenolate mofetil, and a calcineurin inhibitor [1]. These medications all have side effects (see Table 1), which need to be considered when stabilizing kidney transplantation patients and developing a differential diagnosis.

Because of postsurgical anatomic changes as well as the use of immunosuppressive medications, transplant recipients may not present with the typical signs or symptoms [3]. For example, transplant recipients may not mount a febrile response to community-acquired infections such as pneumonia due to immunosuppression and lack of leukocytes to produce the inflammatory reaction or experience dysuria

Table 1 List of common immunosuppressive medications and their side effect profile

Immunosuppressive medication and side effects		
Glucocorticosteroids	Mycophenolate	Tacrolimus
Hypertension	Abdominal pain	Hyperkalemia
Hyperglycemia/diabetes	Nausea/vomiting/diarrhea	Hypertension
Adrenal suppression	Acute inflammatory syndrome	Diabetes mellitus
Fluid retention/weight gain	Increased infection risk	Thrombotic microangiopathy
Psychiatric disturbances	Lymphoproliferative disorders	Increased infection risk
Increased infection risk		Lymphoproliferative disorders

with a urinary tract infection (UTI) due to the lack of innervation of the kidney allograft. Each sign and symptom experienced by the transplant recipient when ill has a broad differential diagnosis. Fortunately, the initial evaluation for each is similar.

With initial assessment of a kidney transplant patient, as with all other pediatric patients, it is important to gather a full set of vital signs including temperature, blood pressure with an appropriately sized cuff, heart rate, and respiratory rate with oxygen saturation. An afebrile patient may still have an acute infection. Hypertension is commonly found in patients with kidney transplantation and is often asymptomatic [1, 3]. The definition of hypertension for pediatric patients is based on percentiles and varies by sex, age, and height. Hypertension can be due to infections (UTI or other common pediatric infections) or noninfectious etiologies such as renal artery stenosis, recurrence of original kidney disease, or urinary obstruction. See Table 2 for a comprehensive list of differential diagnoses for patients presenting with hypertension. Tachycardia may indicate pain, hypovolemia, or compensation for impending shock due to infectious etiology. One important vital sign that may not otherwise be initially considered in pediatric patients is the patient's weight. Transplant recipients are more sensitive to fluid shifts and may have more noticeable weight fluctuations when experiencing illness. Parents will often know the patient's baseline blood pressure or weight; however, if not, it may be helpful to contact the patient's primary nephrologist.

In addition to vital signs, the physical exam can help elucidate the etiology of patient's symptoms. Most kidney transplant recipients retain their native kidneys. The transplant graft is usually located in the right or left lower abdominal quadrant. This is important to note when palpating the abdomen as graft pain may be located in the abdomen or referred to the costovertebral angle. Graft pain may indicate acute infection, rejection, or glucocorticoid immunosuppressive medication side effect. Edema may indicate hypervolemia, salt retention, or nephrotic syndrome. Edema is usually located in dependent areas, which may include lower extremities and periorbital area following sleep. Rashes may be present in the setting of certain infections or graft-versus-host disease.

As described in the patient case presented in this chapter, diarrhea is a common chief complaint among pediatric patients. In the general public, it is usually a

Table 2 Differential diagnosis for pediatric transplant patients presenting with hypertension

Differential diagnosis of hypertension in pediatric transplant patients		
Medications	Vascular/surgical	Other
Steroids	Renal artery stenosis	Pain
Calcineurin inhibitors—cyclosporine, tacrolimus	Renal vein thrombosis	Donor kidney with HTN
	Urine obstruction	Recurrence of original kidney disease
		Failing native kidneys
		Acute infection

self-limiting viral infectious process. In kidney transplant patients, diarrhea can lead to severe dehydration or can represent a more sinister infection. Providers must consider viral and bacterial causes of diarrhea, including more uncommon viral infections such as cytomegalovirus (CMV), norovirus, rotavirus, and BK virus as well as bacterial causes such as *C. difficile* colitis, campylobacter, and *Escherichia coli*. In addition to infectious etiologies of diarrhea, diarrhea alone can indicate rejection, immunosuppressant medication side effect, or even toxicity. Table 3 has a comprehensive list of differential diagnoses of patients with diarrhea. Dehydration in kidney transplant patients can lead to poor perfusion of the kidney graft, which in turn causes elevated creatinine, poor clearance of immunosuppressive medications, and higher risk for toxicity of these medications [3]. Tacrolimus toxicity is a well-documented complication of persistent diarrhea. It is important to attempt to maintain euvolemia during aggressive fluid resuscitation for kidney transplant patients.

In the community hospital setting, the initial evaluation for pediatric kidney transplant patients should include a full set of vitals and a weight. Initial laboratory evaluation should include the following electrolytes: sodium, potassium, chloride, bicarbonate, phosphorus, magnesium, and glucose. Additionally, a BUN and creatinine should be obtained. These electrolytes may be grouped as a renal function panel or basic metabolic panel. A urinalysis with a culture should be obtained to rule out a urinary tract infection. For patients with concerning presentations, a blood culture may also be obtained. Stool studies are not often ordered in the general pediatric patient with diarrhea, but in the patient with a solid-organ transplant, stool cultures may be helpful in identifying an infectious etiology to rule out immunosuppressant medication side effects. Obtaining immunosuppressant medication levels is often not needed in the community setting, especially if patients are to be transferred to higher acuity setting. In most cases, no immediate imaging is necessary in a pediatric transplant patient with diarrhea and/or elevated blood pressure. However, if the creatinine is elevated, one may want to obtain renal transplant ultrasound to rule out any type of urinary obstruction.

The initial management of the 8-year-old boy presented in the case above would include the evaluation discussed above and fluid resuscitation. He is at high risk for dehydration and injury to the graft. Normal saline is the preferred isotonic solution to be used for fluid resuscitation. Extra potassium found in other isotonic fluids such as lactated ringer may be inadequately excreted by an already hypoperfused kidney

Table 3 Differential diagnosis for chief complaint of diarrhea in pediatric transplant patients

Differential diagnosis of diarrhea in pediatric transplant patients		
Infectious	Medication side effect	Other
Bacterial: *C. difficile*, *Campylobacter*, *Salmonella*, *E. coli*, bacterial overgrowth	Immunosuppressants: mycophenolate, tacrolimus, cyclosporine, sirolimus	PTLD, GVHD, malabsorption
Viral: CMV, norovirus, rotavirus, adenovirus	Non-immunosuppressants: antibiotics, proton pump inhibitors, laxatives	
Parasitic: *Giardia*, *Cryptosporidium*, *Entamoeba*		

graft. Similarly, nonsteroidal anti-inflammatory drugs (NSAIDs) should be avoided in kidney transplant patients as they lead to constriction of the afferent arteriole, which causes decreased glomerular filtration rate (GFR) and further damage to the graft. As with the general pediatric population presenting with diarrhea, avoid the use of antispasmodic agents as they can make an infectious diarrhea worse by inhibiting the removal of the offending microorganism. Finally, depending on the estimated glomerular filtration rate of the patient, which may be elevated due to acute kidney injury, medications for symptom management may need to be renally dosed.

6 Review Questions

1. Which of the following measurements is most critical to obtain during the initial management of patients with a kidney transplant?
   (A) Height
   (B) Weight
   (C) Head circumference
   (D) Body mass index
2. Which medications should be avoided in patients with a history of kidney transplantation?
   (A) Acetaminophen
   (B) Nonsteroidal anti-inflammatory drugs
   (C) Morphine
   (D) All of the above
3. Which isotonic fluid should be used for bolus fluid resuscitation in patients with kidney transplantation?
   (A) Normal saline
   (B) Normal saline with dextrose
   (C) Lactated ringer
   (D) PlasmaLyte

7 Answers

1. **B**. In pediatrics, growth charts are important to consider depending on the chief complaint of the presenting patient. For patients with kidney transplantation, weight is an important vital sign to consider. Patients with kidney transplantation are more sensitive to fluid shifts. For example, patients with a history of kidney transplantation may have increased weight from the use of steroids or rejection of graft. Weight loss may occur more readily when patients are experiencing dehydration or hypovolemic shock.

2. **B**. As with the adult population, pediatric patients may present with pain. Pain is notoriously undertreated in the pediatric population. Providers should avoid the use of NSAIDs in patients with kidney transplantation due to the risk of afferent arteriole constriction leading to acute kidney injury, which can damage the kidney graph. Acetaminophen is cleared by the liver and is a safe alternative for pain control. If acetaminophen is not sufficient, appropriate doses of opioid medications may be used for pain when warranted. Caution must be taken when using morphine in patients with severe AKI as the metabolites may accumulate and cause neurologic symptoms.
3. **A.** Normal saline is the appropriate isotonic solution to use as initial fluid resuscitation for patients with kidney disease. Dosing is 20 mL/kg. Dextrose may be used if the patient is hypoglycemic; however, using normal saline with dextrose is not an appropriate isotonic solution for all treatment of dehydration as it may lead to hyperglycemia. Lactated ringer contains 4 mEq/L of potassium. In patients with kidney transplantation, potassium supplementation should be avoided as it may be poorly excreted in the setting of AKI. Similarly, PlasmaLyte is a balanced isotonic solution containing 5 mEq/L of potassium and should not be used in patients with kidney transplantation.

8 Takeaway Points

1. Kidney transplantation complications may include acute, subacute, and chronic conditions, which range across surgical complications, infectious complications, or medication side effects.
2. Vital signs, including weight, may be abnormal in patients with kidney transplant as these patients often are on immunosuppressant medications.
3. Providers should include common pediatric community-acquired etiologies of symptoms as well as those unique to transplant patients in the differential diagnosis.

   Initial evaluation should include serum electrolytes, serum creatinine, and urinalysis. Imaging is often not needed on first-pass evaluation unless there is specific concern for urinary obstruction.
4. Initial management should include aggressive fluid resuscitation with normal saline and avoidance of medications that may worsen acute kidney injuries such as NSAIDs and potassium-containing solutions.

References

1. Saeed B. Pediatric renal transplantation. Int J Organ Transplant Med. 2012;3(2):62–73.
2. Dharnidkharka VR, Fiorina P, Harmon WE. Kidney transplantation in children. N Engl J Med. 2014;371:549–58. https://doi.org/10.1056/NEJMra1314376.

3. Winterberg PD, Garro R. Long-term outcomes of kidney transplantation in children. Pediatr Clin N Am. 2019;66(1):269–80. https://doi.org/10.1016/j.pcl.2018.09.008.
4. OPTN National Data Report, Kidney Transplants by Recipient Age, retrieved 10/09/2023 from https://optn.transplant.hrsa.gov/data/view-data-reports/national-data/#.
5. Jorgensen DR, Wu CM, Hariharan S. Epidemiology of end-stage renal failure among twins and diagnosis, management, and current outcomes of kidney transplantation between identical twins. Am J Transplant. 2020;20(3):761–8. https://doi.org/10.1111/ajt.15638. Epub 2019 Nov 5.

A Patient with a Liver Transplant and Abdominal Pain

Stacey Stauber, Esther Jun-Ihn, and Robert Venick

1 Case

An 18-year-old boy with a history of biliary atresia status post orthotopic liver transplant at 1 year of age presents with right upper quadrant (RUQ) abdominal pain and fever for 2 days. The patient reports feeling otherwise well until 2 days ago when he developed fevers up to 102°F with minimal relief of symptoms despite taking acetaminophen. The same day, he developed intermittent, sharp, RUQ pain with no radiation. He rates the pain 6–9/10. He does note that he has been feeling tired over the past week with nasal congestion and rhinorrhea and no cough. He has also been complaining of chills, headache, pruritus, and yellowing of his eyes. He has no vomiting or diarrhea and no sick contacts. He has enrolled in summer online classes. He endorses taking his medication regularly with a few missed doses per week. His parents are not always present when taking medications because they are working. Overall, he has been doing well the past 17 years with no major complications after his initial surgery.

On exam, he is febrile to 38.5°F and slightly tachycardic with all other vitals within normal limits. Your physical exam is notable for a patient in mild discomfort with scleral icterus, tachycardia without any murmurs, and a soft and non-distended abdomen with tenderness to palpation of the RUQ. He exhibits normal mentation. No petechiae or bruising is noted.

S. Stauber · E. Jun-Ihn (✉) · R. Venick
Department of Pediatrics, UCLA Mattel Children's Hospital, Los Angeles, CA, USA
e-mail: SStauber@mednet.ucla.edu; EJun@mednet.ucla.edu; RVenick@mednet.ucla.edu

A. Kamzan et al. (eds.), *Children with Medical Complexity in the Emergency Department*, https://doi.org/10.1007/978-3-031-62517-6_20

2 Discussion Questions

1. What empiric antibiotic coverage would be recommended with this patient's presentation?
2. Besides transplant rejection, what is on your initial differential diagnosis?
3. What are the appropriate initial studies based on the patient's presentation?

3 Case Answers

1. Initial antibiotics should include coverage for anaerobic and gram-negative organisms with a fourth-generation cephalosporin + metronidazole or piperacillin-tazobactam given concern for acute cholangitis on presentation. Infection is the number one cause of death in liver transplant recipients, so it is important to treat urgently [1].
2. High on the initial differential besides transplant rejection is infection including acute cholangitis, community-acquired infections, and viral opportunistic infections like Epstein-Barr virus (EBV) viremia and cytomegalovirus (CMV) viremia. Of note, infection with subsequent immune stimulation is a common risk factor for developing acute rejection.
3. Initial preliminary studies should include total and direct bilirubin, ALT, AST, GGT, EBV/CMV quantitative serum PCRs, bacterial culture (consider fungal culture), and immunosuppressant blood levels. Ultrasound of liver with Doppler can be a good screening test to assess for late surgical complications such as hepatic artery thrombosis, portal vein thrombosis, inferior vena cava/hepatic vein stenosis, and biliary strictures.

4 Learning Objectives

1. Recognize common causes of acute liver transplant rejection.
2. Describe the initial workup and management of acute liver transplant rejection.
3. Recognize late complications of children with liver transplants.

5 Discussion

Providers who take care of pediatric transplant patients must remain vigilant to the broad differential diagnosis in patients presenting with acute symptoms. Fevers may be a sign of infection, acute rejection of the transplanted organ, or malignancy such as PTLD (post-transplant lymphoproliferative disorder). Patients who have undergone a liver transplant are at a higher risk of infections given their need for lifelong immunosuppressive therapy [1, 2].

As mentioned above, patients with liver transplants are at increased risk of infections including bacterial, fungal, and opportunistic infections such as EBV and CMV viremia. These patients may present with fever and/or signs of graft dysfunction including elevated transaminases, jaundice, or pruritus. Infections can occur at any point in the lifetime of a transplant recipient. Certain infections are more common in the initial postoperative period related to surgery itself and foreign bodies such as central venous catheters and drains, while infections months to years posttransplant may be related to immunosuppression and opportunistic infections [3].

Acute rejection can be precipitated by medication nonadherence, difficulty obtaining stable immunosuppression levels, and infections. Given this patient's adolescent age and transitioning of medical supervision from parents to self, it is important to consider possible medication nonadherence and acute rejection as a part of his presentation. It is important to recognize rejection as it can precipitate graft loss if not appropriately treated. Acute rejection is often T-cell mediated and usually responds to pulse steroids as well as an increase in maintenance immunosuppression. Antibody-mediated rejection as well as chronic rejection, on the other hand, can be more challenging to treat and may lead to re-transplantation [1, 2].

One must keep malignancy on the differential in transplant patients presenting with fevers. One malignancy, in particular, that is always important to keep in mind with liver transplant patients is PTLD. Patients do not always present with lymphadenopathy. PTLD occurs in up to 2–15% of pediatric liver transplant recipients [3]. Liver transplant recipients who are EBV negative but receive an EBV-positive transplant are at higher risk of seroconversion or primary EBV infection. EBV PCRs are monitored closely posttransplant. PTLD treatment includes immunosuppression reduction. Patients may also need rituximab and/or chemotherapy [3].

The best laboratory indicators for acute liver rejection are elevation in bilirubin, AST and ALT, GGT, and alkaline phosphatase as well as low immunosuppressant levels. Cultures, both bacterial and fungal, are important to rule out infections as described above. These labs can also be elevated in the setting of infections or other liver injury, so histologic evidence with a liver biopsy is important for diagnosis of rejection. The treatment of acute rejection usually consists of pulse steroids and an increase in maintenance immunosuppression [1, 2]. Acute rejection needs to be treated urgently and managed appropriately given that it can lead to graft loss if not appropriately treated in a timely manner. As in the above case, adolescence is a well-documented, high-risk time for nonadherence with medications, leading to low immunosuppressant levels potentiating late acute rejection [2].

Additional causes of poor graft function are late surgical complications, most commonly hepatic artery thrombosis. Other late surgical complications include portal venous thrombosis, inferior vena cava/hepatic vein stenosis, and biliary strictures [2, 3]. Additional laboratory findings in late surgical complications include anemia from splenomegaly or varices or hypoalbuminemia from portal venous thrombosis leading to ascites and protein-losing enteropathy. First-line screening imaging for these complications is typically Doppler ultrasound examination of the liver. Ultrasound examination would assess for the hepatic vessel vasculature as well as biliary strictures, biliary abscess, and liver texture/size. Other imaging options include computed tomography (CT) or magnetic resonance (MR) with contrast, and more advanced imaging modalities include combination MR angiogram combined to MR cholangiopancreatography (MRCP). If biliary strictures are noted on any of the aforementioned testing, more invasive examinations may include endoscopic retrograde cholangiopancreatography (ERCP) or percutaneous transhepatic cholangiogram (PTC) to actively place a biliary stent or drain for biliary strictures after careful examination of the hepatic vessels. Poor graft function due to recurrence of primary liver disease in children is an infrequent finding, although this occurs more frequently in adult recipients transplanted for nonalcoholic fatty liver disease, hepatitis C, alcohol-associated liver disease, viral hepatitis, autoimmune hepatitis, and sclerosing cholangitis [3].

Given the risk of intra-abdominal infections such as cholangitis, coverage for anaerobic organisms and gram-negative organisms such as *Enterobacter* and *Pseudomonas* remains the mainstay for initial antibiotic treatment. Examples of appropriate empiric antibiotics include cefepime plus metronidazole or monotherapy with either piperacillin-tazobactam or meropenem. These antibiotics are generally well tolerated by patients with liver transplants without the need for laboratory monitoring when used for short courses.

For those patients who continue to require a central line (for intravenous medications posttransplant or extremely difficult access with need for frequent lab draws), it is important to cover for gram-positive organisms such as *Staphylococcus* in addition to the anaerobic and gram-negative organisms mentioned above. Vancomycin is often the initial antibiotic used but requires frequent monitoring and should be used with caution in children who have undergone a liver transplant given that their immunosuppressive medications can be nephrotoxic. These children have a higher risk of chronic kidney disease even if their creatinine and estimated GFR appear normal [2]. Immunosuppressive medications can contribute to de novo acute and chronic posttransplant renal dysfunction. The cumulative 5-year incidence of chronic renal failure among adult liver transplant recipients is about 18% [3]. Linezolid is an option if vancomycin is contraindicated, but it should be used with caution in patients with baseline cytopenias as linezolid could worsen blood dyscrasias.

For this patient in the above case, without a central line but concerns for cholangitis with fever and RUQ pain, piperacillin-tazobactam would be an appropriate first-line agent to start empirically (Table 1).

Table 1 Acute liver transplant rejection presentation and workup

Clinical signs	Labs	Imaging	Management
• Hepatosplenomegaly • RUQ abdominal pain • Pruritus • Scleral icterus • Changes in stool consistency and color	• LFTs • Total bilirubin and direct bilirubin • PT/INR • EBV and CMV PCRs • Bacterial blood cultures	Liver ultrasound with duplex	Start piperacillin-tazobactam Admission to transplant center to assess for rejection with liver biopsy

6 Review Questions

1. What is the gold standard for diagnosis of liver transplant rejection?
   (A) Laboratory findings of transaminitis and elevated GGT
   (B) MR elastography to assess for liver fibrosis
   (C) Percutaneous liver biopsy
   (D) Endoscopic retrograde cholangiopancreatography
2. What is the initial management for acute liver transplant rejection?
   (A) Re-transplantation
   (B) Bolus doses of steroids
   (C) Switching immunosuppression from tacrolimus to cyclosporine
   (D) Anti-interleukin-2 receptor monoclonal antibody treatment
3. What are the important risk factors for acute rejection?
   (A) Recipient age >13 years of age
   (B) Tacrolimus immunosuppression
   (C) Asian descent
   (D) Living donor organ

7 Answers

1. **C**. A liver biopsy is the standard of practice to diagnosis acute rejection. Elevated AST/ALT and GGT are not specific enough to diagnose rejection, and MR elastography to assess for liver fibrosis is being studied in children with cystic fibrosis and nonalcoholic liver disease. ERCP or PTC would be helpful if there was any concern for biliary stricture and would allow for the placement of a biliary stent but cannot be utilized to diagnose rejection.
2. **B**. Most children with acute rejection will respond to pulse steroids and increased calcineurin inhibitor levels, most commonly tacrolimus. Additional immunosuppressants that have been successful as adjunct therapy to treating rejection include mycophenolate and mTOR inhibitors in combination with calcineurin inhibitors. Tacrolimus has markedly reduced the incidence of chronic rejection compared to cyclosporine. Anti-interleukin-2 receptor monoclonal antibody treatment has been found to be successful during induction therapy in order to prevent acute rejection 7–10 days after transplant surgery but is not the best initial treatment for acute rejection. Re-transplantation is a consideration for poor response to treatment but would not be initially considered.
3. **A**. In a large North American study of 38 liver transplant centers, recipient age <13 years old, living-related donors, and tacrolimus immunosuppression experienced lower rates of rejection [1]. Children under 6 months of age have the lowest rate of rejection [1]. Patients on tacrolimus have lower rates of rejection

compared to those on cyclosporine. African American descent has been found to have higher rates of rejection. Adolescence is a major risk factor for medication nonadherence. Successful transition to adult care is recommended between 18 and 23 years and requires years of multidisciplinary education and preparation by the pediatric transplant team. Suboptimal transition process has an increased risk of nonadherence and graft loss. Parents need to encourage and promote patient independence. Additional resources for transitioning are available at the Pediatric Transition Portal by the American Society of Transplantation.

8 Takeaway Points

1. Initial clinical management for pediatric liver transplant recipients with fevers and transaminitis includes hepatic function panel, GGT, cultures, liver ultrasound with Doppler, and IV antibiotics with anaerobic and gram-negative antibiotic coverage.
2. Initial diagnostic considerations for pediatric liver transplant recipients with fevers and transaminitis: rejection (acute vs. chronic), biliary strictures with associated cholangitis, hepatic artery thrombosis, portal vein thrombosis, PTLD, and infection.
3. We strongly recommend transfer to a specialized transplantation center when there is concern for rejection or late postsurgical complications, a need for urgent liver biopsy, and additional advanced imaging and interventions.

References

1. Martin SR, Atkison P, Anand R, Lindblad AS. Studies of Pediatric Liver Transplantation 2002: patient and graft survival and rejection in pediatric recipients of a first liver transplant in the United States and Canada. Pediatr Transplant. 2004;8:273–83. https://doi.org/10.1111/j.1399-3046.2004.00152.x.
2. Kelly DA, Bucuvalas JC, Alonso EM, Karpen SJ, Allen U, Green M, Farmer D, Shemesh E, McDonald RA. Long-term medical management of the pediatric patient after liver transplantation: 2013 practice guideline by the American Association for the Study of Liver Diseases and the American Society of Transplantation. Liver Transplant. 2013;19(8):798–825. https://doi.org/10.1002/lt.23697.
3. McGuire BM, Rosenthal P, Brown CC, Busch AM, Calcatera SM, Claria RS, Hunt NK, Korenblat KM, Mazariegos GV, Moonka D, Orloff SL, Perry DK, Rosen CB, Scott DL, Sudan DL, American Society of Transplantation. Long-term management of the liver transplant patient: recommendations for the primary care doctor. Am J Transplant. 2009;9(9):1988–2003. https://doi.org/10.1111/j.1600-6143.2009.02733.x. Epub 2009 Jun 26.

Increased Ostomy Output and Fevers in a Child with Small Bowel Transplant

Esther Jun-Ihn, Stacey Stauber, and Robert Venick

1 Case

A 4-year-old female with a history of gastroschisis complicated by bowel necrosis and perforation requiring extensive bowel resection resulting in short gut syndrome with intestinal failure and liver disease (IFALD) status post combined liver, intestinal, and pancreas transplant last year presents with increased ostomy output for the past week and fevers for 1 day.

The parents noticed that the ostomy output has been consistently more watery as well as increased in volume with worsening edema of her ostomy site. For the past month or so, the volume has been intermittently high, but over the past week, it has been consistently high volume. The stool is loose, yellow-brown in color, with no obvious blood. Typically, her outputs are ~25 ml/kg/day with thicker consistency, but in the last week, the parents measured greater than 40 ml/kg/day. Fevers started this afternoon, with a maximum temperature of 38.5 °C. There has been no cough, sore throat, nausea, vomiting, or abdominal pain. She does have sick contacts, which is her younger brother with diarrhea for the past day. There has been no recent travel. She is tolerating food by mouth and 4–4.5 cartons of Peptamen Junior daily via her gastrostomy tube overnight.

The patient started school a few months ago. She still has a central line in place for intermittent intravenous (IV) hydration and labs. Her parents have been flushing the catheter daily with no issues.

On exam, the patient is well-appearing with a temperature of 38.3°C and in no acute distress. Additional vitals were in normal range except for tachycardia of 146. Her lungs are clear to auscultation. She has generalized abdominal pain, but

E. Jun-Ihn (✉) · S. Stauber · R. Venick
Department of Pediatrics, UCLA Mattel Children's Hospital, Los Angeles, CA, USA
e-mail: EJun@mednet.ucla.edu; SStauber@mednet.ucla.edu; RVenick@mednet.ucla.edu

A. Kamzan et al. (eds.), *Children with Medical Complexity in the Emergency Department*, https://doi.org/10.1007/978-3-031-62517-6_21

normoactive bowel sounds. She has well-healed abdominal surgical scars. The output in ostomy bag is watery and light brown. The stoma site is erythematous with slight bleeding. A gastrostomy tube is in place. A central line site on the right chest is clean, dry, and intact with no drainage with inspection and palpation.

2 Discussion Questions

1. What are the signs of acute rejection in children with small bowel transplants (SBTs)?
2. What are the important initial resuscitation and access concerns in children with SBTs that are unique compared to other solid-organ transplants?
3. What is the most common post-transplant complication associated with children with SBTs?

3 Case Answers

1. Clinical signs of acute rejection in children with SBTs are nonspecific, including high ostomy output, bloody diarrhea, generalized abdominal pain, and fevers.
2. Patients typically have limited enteral absorption from underlying disease, and all resuscitative medications should be given IV as much as possible. It is also important to closely follow electrolytes given poor intestinal absorption.
3. Sepsis is the most frequent cause of mortality, including bacterial, viral, and fungal infections, primarily from their central venous catheter and intra-abdominal sources.

4 Learning Objectives

1. Clinical signs of rejection in children with SBTs.
2. Common causes of acute rejection in children with SBTs.
3. Initial workup and management of acute rejection for children with SBTs.

5 Discussion

Of the solid-organ transplants, intestinal transplantation is least frequent, likely due to higher morbidity and mortality. The intestines are very immunoreactive given the large lymphoid tissue transplanted with the small bowel, thus making 1-year graft survival lower than children with other solid-organ transplants [1]. Overall survival continues to improve due to an increase in 1-year graft survival from optimization of immunosuppression and improved surgical techniques.

There are many indications for intestinal transplant; however, given the continued high morbidity and mortality, intestinal transplant is often reserved for patients with progressive intestinal failure, recurrent episodes of sepsis with organ dysfunction, loss of central venous access, poor quality of life, and congenital mucosal disorders [1, 2]. The most common indication for intestinal transplant is intestinal failure like the case. Many of the conditions leading to intestinal failure arise from congenital and neonatal conditions, including short gut syndromes from congenital atresias, gastroschisis, malrotation with volvulus, surgical resections from necrotizing enterocolitis, and trauma. Less common congenital conditions include motility disorders such as long-segment Hirschsprung's disease, intestinal pseudo-obstruction, and enteropathies such as congenital diarrhea syndrome, microvillous inclusion disease, and tufting enteropathy among others as well [1].

Given the higher immunogenicity of the intestines, there is a higher likelihood of acute and chronic rejection. Early signs of acute rejection in children with SBTs include higher than normal ostomy output, bloody ostomy output, abdominal pain, and fever. Like other organ transplants, recognizing the signs of acute rejection promptly is crucial for graft and patient survival. Typical ostomy output can be as high as 30 ml/kg/day given the lack of the large intestines to help retain water. Unlike elevated b-type natriuretic peptide (BNP) in heart transplant patients or elevated liver enzymes in liver transplant recipients, there is no reliable blood or noninvasive biomarker to assess for acute rejection in SBTs. There are a few biomarkers that are being used by transplant centers such as plasma citrulline (made by enterocytes), fecal calprotectin which can be elevated in the stool with active inflammation (but it does not differentiate between rejection, graft-versus-host disease (GVHD), infection, and posttransplant lymphoproliferative disorder (PTLD)), and reg-3 alpha (regenerating islet-derived 3-alpha expressed by gastrointestinal epithelium) with elevation from gastrointestinal mucosal injury [1].

Although high ostomy output, fever, and abdominal pain should raise clinical suspicion for acute rejection, infection or PTLD are additional diagnoses to consider. In up to 50% of patients, sepsis can lead to death [1]. Causes of sepsis include viral, bacterial, and fungal sources, which can lead to graft dysfunction. Enterococcus species are a frequently isolated bacterial organism, but other sources of sepsis include cytomegalovirus (CMV), adenovirus, and Epstein-Barr virus (EBV).

When children with SBTs present with concerns for acute rejection and fevers, it is important to establish IV access immediately, given the concern for sepsis. As previously mentioned, sepsis is the most frequent cause of death after transplantation, and often these children have limited antibiotic sensitivities and should be started on broader antibiotics than other organ recipients [1, 2]. Common bacterial organisms to cover include gram-positive bacteria, gram-negative (like *Pseudomonas*) bacteria, and anaerobic bacteria. Broad-spectrum antibiotics to empirically start include piperacillin/tazobactam or meropenem. It is also important to consider adding MRSA coverage with vancomycin, for example, if there are any retained lines or drains like a central venous catheter. Children who receive SBTs or combined intestinal, liver, and pancreas transplants are also at higher risk for fungal and viral infections given that they require a higher dose of immunosuppression than other solid-organ transplants [1]. Consider adding empiric antifungal coverage with caspofungin, for example, if children present particularly ill. Given that these children are also at risk for viral illnesses, it is also helpful in the initial screen to obtain not only bacterial and fungal blood cultures, but also viral serum PCRs for CMV, EBV, and adenovirus. Stool studies are also routinely sent given the increase in ostomy output to assess for bacterial enteric pathogens, *Clostridium difficile*, rotavirus, norovirus, adenovirus, and *Enterovirus*, among others.

Children with SBTs also typically have limited enteral absorption, and all resuscitative medications should be given IV if possible. It is also important to closely follow electrolytes given the poor intestinal reabsorption. Given higher stool outputs, patients might also benefit from more fluids that provide stool replacement like sodium acetate or albumin for adequate fluid optimization. Also, it is important to monitor the hemoglobin closely with a complete blood count (CBC) given that these children can produce bloody ostomy output from ulcerative mucosa and a disrupted epithelial barrier. While the patient in the case already had central venous access, children with SBTs often have significantly limited central venous access sites [1]. If additional central access is required, children will need to be evaluated urgently at a small bowel transplant center.

The diagnosis of acute rejection (ACR) in these patients is a combination of clinical, endoscopic, and histologic parameters [1, 2]. The gold standard of diagnosis is intestinal biopsies. If there is a concern for rejection, these children should be transferred urgently to an SBT center for intestinal biopsies. To effectively screen for ACR, given the lack of biomarkers, these patients are often left with an ileostomy to have access for frequent biopsies. If ileal biopsies show no evidence of rejection, another intervention to consider is an upper endoscopy with proximal small bowel biopsies. Mucosal changes in rejection often parallel Acute rejection (ACR) Small bowel transplantation (SBT) the severity of intestinal injury with common findings including edema, focal erosions, or ulcerations [3]. Other findings on histology that are consistent with acute rejection include inflammatory infiltrates and crypt apoptosis [3]. Biopsies can also be assessed for viral testing on the tissue and histological evaluation. Treatment for ACR should be started promptly. Rejection remains the primary cause of graft loss in these patients. Mild to moderate ACR can be controlled with pulse steroids and increasing immunosuppression, but patients with moderate to severe ACR may need antithymocyte globulin and additional immunomodulators [1, 2]. While patients are receiving treatment for ACR, they may need further supportive care, such as converting all medications to IV, starting parenteral nutrition, and continuing additional fluid replacement with either sodium acetate or albumin for elevated ostomy output >30 ml/kg/day.

6 Review Questions

1. What is the most common cause of intestinal failure in children?
   (A) Re-transplantation
   (B) Short bowel syndrome
   (C) Motility disorders
   (D) Malabsorption
2. What is the gold standard for diagnosis of acute rejection in children with SBTs?
   (A) Upper gastrointestinal imaging with small bowel follow-through
   (B) Endoscopic findings from upper endoscopy and ileoscopy
   (C) Histologic findings from intestinal biopsy
   (D) Magnetic resonance (MR) enterography
3. After the initial resuscitation of children with SBTs, what additional fluids are important to start?
   (A) IV ostomy or stool replacement fluid
   (B) Enteral fluids
   (C) Oral fluids to prevent loss of oral autonomy
   (D) No additional fluids are needed
4. What are the best antibiotics to empirically start when children with SBTs and central venous catheters present with concerns for sepsis and acute rejection?
   (A) Ceftriaxone and linezolid
   (B) Caspofungin and vancomycin
   (C) Piperacillin/tazobactam and vancomycin
   (D) Ceftriaxone and metronidazole

7 Answers

1. **B**. Short bowel syndrome is the leading cause of intestinal failure comprising 63% of children who meet the criteria for intestinal transplantation. Short bowel syndrome is defined as a small bowel length of <25 cm without an ileocecal valve. It typically arises from neonatal conditions such as gastroschisis, intestinal volvulus, intestinal atresia, and necrotizing enterocolitis [1].
2. **C**. Gold standard for diagnosis of acute rejection in SBT recipients is histologic findings on biopsy from either ileoscopy or upper endoscopy. Endoscopic findings are helpful in characterizing any areas of ulceration or loss of vasculature, but the pathologic criteria of acute rejection are based on histologic findings. Imaging can be obtained in the initial management of acute rejection but cannot be utilized to diagnose rejection.

3. **A**. It is important to start IV ostomy or stool replacement with either sodium acetate or albumin for ostomy output >30 cc/kg/day given their high output. Enteral and oral fluids would not be sufficient given the lack of intestinal absorption during acute rejection.
4. **C**. Children with SBTs need broader coverage for antimicrobials when they present in sepsis given their lack of intestinal absorption and limited antibiotic sensitivity. It is important to empirically cover for gram-positive, gram-negative, and anaerobic organisms. Antifungal coverage can be considered, but caspofungin and vancomycin do not have sufficient bacterial coverage. Central venous catheter and intra-abdominal sources are the most common causes of sepsis.

8 Takeaway Points

1. Rejection in children with SBTs is more clinically ambiguous than other organ recipients, and there is no reliable biomarker to assess for it.
2. Children with SBTs who present with clinical concerns for acute rejection should be aggressively treated with appropriate IV antibiotics and fluids and transferred to a transplant center to assess for rejection via intestinal biopsies.
3. Sepsis is the leading cause of mortality in these children, and they often need broader coverage with antimicrobials given their limited antibiotic sensitivity and poor enteral absorption.

References

1. Martinez Rivera A, Wales PW. Intestinal transplantation in children: current status. Pediatr Surg Int. 2016;32(6):529–40. https://doi.org/10.1007/s00383-016-3885-2. Epub 2016 Mar 31.
2. Raghu VK, Beaumont JL, Everly MJ, Venick RS, Lacaille F, Mazariegos GV. Pediatric intestinal transplantation: analysis of the intestinal transplant registry. Pediatr Transplant. 2019;23(8):e13580. https://doi.org/10.1111/petr.13580. Epub 2019 Sep 18.
3. Narang A, Dong X, Mitsinikos T, Genyk Y, Thomas D, Kohli R, Lin C-H, Soufi N, Warren M, Merritt R, Yanni G. Severe late-onset acute cellular rejection in a pediatric patient with isolated small intestinal transplant rescued with aggressive immunosuppressive approach: a case report. Transplant Proc. 2019;51(9):3181–5. https://doi.org/10.1016/j.transproceed.2019.08.012.

A Complication of Polypharmacy

Shahram Yazdani, Pauline Yi, and Vidhi Doshi

1 Case

A 12-year-old patient was transported by law enforcement to the emergency department for headache, nausea, agitation, fever, and sweating that started 3 hours ago. The infirmary physician was concerned about the sudden onset and severity of her symptoms. Her physical exam is significant for heart rate of 143, blood pressure of 150/100, and shallow breathing. Her past medical history is significant for cyclic vomiting syndrome, migraines, and a ventricular septal defect. She recently started treatment for ADHD and depression. Officers cannot rule out any ingestion or suicidal attempts.

2 Discussion Questions

1. What is the most urgent etiology to be considered?
2. What is the best treatment for this condition?

S. Yazdani (✉)
Department of Pediatrics, University of California, Los Angeles, CA, USA
e-mail: syazdani@mednet.ucla.edu

P. Yi · V. Doshi
Department of Medicine, University of California, Los Angeles, CA, USA
e-mail: pyi@mednet.ucla.edu; vdoshi@mednet.ucla.edu

A. Kamzan et al. (eds.), *Children with Medical Complexity in the Emergency Department*, https://doi.org/10.1007/978-3-031-62517-6_22

3 Case Answers

1. Given the patient's sudden onset of symptoms including headache, nausea, agitation, fever, and sweating, along with significant vital sign abnormalities, the most serious and urgent diagnosis to be considered is serotonin syndrome. The interaction between the amphetamines used in ADHD treatment and depression medications (e.g., serotonin reuptake inhibitors) in this patient can cause serotonin syndrome. Some treatments for migraines and cyclic vomiting syndrome may also increase the risk. It is also concerning that there is a possibility of ingestion or suicidal attempts, which can further complicate the clinical picture.
2. Treatment typically involves discontinuing the suspected medications, providing supportive care, and, in severe cases, admission to intensive care unit for hemodynamic support, pharmacologic treatment, and mechanical ventilation.

4 Learning Objectives

1. Understand the various categories of adverse drug reactions.
2. Recognize the risks of polypharmacy, particularly for children with medical complexity.
3. Describe the management of common adverse drug reactions.

5 Discussion

Adverse drug reactions (ADRs) represent a significant risk factor in hospitalized children. Children with medical complexities that are treated with multiple medications are at increased risk of developing ADR due to drug interactions and their fragile state of health.

5.1 Neurologic Complications of Medications in Medically Complex Children

The neurologic subtypes of ADR may range from mild to potentially life-threatening conditions. Seizure, tardive dyskinesia, serotonin syndrome, drug-induced diabetes insipidus, neuroleptic malignant syndrome, and posterior reversible encephalopathy syndrome represent some of the most serious and potentially life-threatening ADRs, while headaches, dizziness, nausea, and vomiting represent some of the more common and benign reactions. The following table represents the list of neurologic reactions and causative agents (Table 1) [1].

Table 1 Neurologic symptoms of adverse drug reactions

Symptom	Drugs associated
Ataxia	Anticholinergic agents, antiepileptic drugs, anticancer agents, sedatives, hypnotics, lithium, cyclosporine, nitrous oxide, alcohol, and recreational drugs like ketamine and dextromethorphan
Dysarthria	Anticancer agents, phenytoin, aripiprazole, benzodiazepines, lithium, neuroleptic drugs, and paroxetine
Dysphagia	Anticholinergic agents, antipsychotics, muscle relaxants, phenytoin toxicity, sedative/hypnotics/narcotics
Falls	Anticholinergic, antidepressants (e.g., nortriptyline, venlafaxine), antiepileptic, antipsychotics (olanzapine), cardiovascular drugs (i.e., beta-blockers, calcium channel blockers, diuretics, renin-angiotensin system inhibitors, and vasodilators), sedative/hypnotics/narcotics
Headaches	Aminophenol derivatives, antihistamines, barbiturates, intravenous immunoglobulin, opioids, salicylates, triptans, antibiotics, antiepileptics, antidepressants, oral contraceptives, sildenafil, vasodilators, immunoglobulins, ondansetron, nicotine
Hearing loss	Antibiotics, antiepileptic drugs, salicylates, antimalarials, antineoplastic agents, diuretics, calcium channel blockers, beta-adrenergic receptor blockers
Hiccups	Alcohol, anesthetics, antibiotics (e.g., beta-lactams, macrolides, and fluoroquinolones), atypical antipsychotics, benzodiazepines, barbiturates, chemotherapy, corticosteroids, opioids, phenytoin, sedatives, selective serotonin reuptake inhibitors, and tricyclic antidepressants
Insomnia	Alcohol, antidepressants, antiepileptic drugs, antihistamines, antimalarials, antineoplastics, bronchodilators, cardiovascular drugs, CNS stimulants, drug withdrawals for opioids, and corticosteroids
Nausea and vomiting	Alcohol, anesthetics, antibiotics, anticonvulsants, chemotherapy agents, nonsteroidal anti-inflammatory drugs, opioids, progesterone, and radiotherapy
Neurologic bladder	Anticholinergic drugs (antimuscarinic, antinicotinic, neuroleptics, and tricyclic antidepressants)
Syncope	Analgesics, antineoplastics drugs, interferon alpha, hypnotic sedative drugs, hypoglycemic drugs, selective serotonin reuptake inhibitors, CNS stimulants, loperamide, sildenafil, vasodilators, antipsychotics, antihypertensives, and topical ophthalmic preparations
Vertigo and dizziness	Alcohol, aminoglycoside antibiotics, anticonvulsants, antidepressants, antihypertensives, barbiturates, benzodiazepines, chemotherapeutic agents, loop diuretics, salicylates, ototoxic drugs, neuroleptics, sedatives, hypoglycemic agents, and opioids
Visual impairment	Antimalarials, antimicrobials, antineoplastics, corticosteroids, GABA-mimetic antiepileptic agents, interferon-alpha, immunosuppressant agents, nonsteroidal anti-inflammatory drugs, and sildenafil

5.1.1 Tardive Dyskinesia (TD)

Tardive dyskinesia (TD) is a rare, medication-induced hyperkinetic movement disorder of neurological origin, predominantly associated with dopamine receptor-blocking agents. This includes first- and second-generation antipsychotic drugs, metoclopramide, and prochlorperazine. These drugs penetrate the blood-brain barrier, potentially inducing abnormal movements in the oro-bucco-lingual region in genetically predisposed individuals, particularly at elevated doses and prolonged durations of use. The timeline for TD onset is variable, ranging from 3 months to several years post-initial drug administration. Clinical manifestations include involuntary movements of the head, face, and tongue such as facial tics, lip smacking, and head nodding. However, the extremities, trunk, and respiratory muscles may also be impacted. In some cases, dystonia may serve as an initial symptom.

Diagnosis of TD can be challenging due to its clinical resemblance to disorders such as autism or Rett syndrome. Prompt identification and cessation of the causative drug can considerably improve the prognosis and shorten the recovery period. Medication withdrawal should ideally be gradual, extending over weeks to months, to avoid exacerbation of TD symptoms. Total resolution of tardive movements may be a prolonged process, extending from months to years after the cessation of the offending drug, with no guarantee of complete recovery. In mild TD cases, discontinuation of the causative medication may not be necessary, and symptoms can be managed with vesicular monoamine transporter type 2 inhibitors (VMAT2) or benzodiazepines. Tetrabenazine, deutetrabenazine, and valbenazine are the VMAT2 medications presently approved in the United States. In adults with severe, treatment-resistant TD, deep brain stimulation may provide symptomatic relief [2].

Given the limited therapeutic options, preventative measures are paramount. These include prescribing the minimal effective dose of second-generation antipsychotics, comprehensive patient education, and vigilant monitoring for potential adverse effects.

5.1.2 Serotonin Syndrome (SS)

Serotonin syndrome is a potentially life-threatening condition characterized by a collection of symptoms including altered mental state, autonomic dysfunctions, neuromuscular hyperactivity, and seizures. Altered mental status may present as agitation, restlessness, and confusion, while the autonomic irregularities may include excessive diaphoresis, rapid heart rate (tachycardia), elevated body temperature (hyperthermia), high blood pressure (hypertension), and gastrointestinal disturbances including vomiting and diarrhea. Neuromuscular hyperactivity may be evident through tremors, involuntary muscle jerks (myoclonus), and heightened reflexes (hyperreflexia).

Serotonin syndrome should be suspected in children who are undergoing treatment by medications that increase serotonin levels in the brain such as selective serotonin reuptake inhibitors, serotonin-norepinephrine reuptake inhibitors, tricyclic antidepressants, anti-migraine medications (e.g., carbamazepine, valproic acid, and triptans), dextromethorphan, and certain pain medications including opioids. Serotonin-norepinephrine reuptake inhibitors are slightly more likely to cause serotonin syndrome compared to selective serotonin reuptake inhibitors. Drugs of abuse such as methylenedioxymethamphetamine (MDMA) may also contribute to serotonin syndrome.

The diagnosis of serotonin syndrome is made solely on clinical grounds, requiring a detailed history and physical, and a comprehensive neurologic examination to differentiate from similarly presenting neurologic or infectious conditions.

The majority of patients with serotonin syndrome require hospital admission and observation, with the most severe cases requiring stabilization and treatment in the intensive care unit. Treatment should begin with stabilization and supportive care, including oxygen, intravenous fluids, and continuous cardiac monitoring. Autonomic instability and hyperthermia require aggressive treatment with serotonergic antagonists such as cyproheptadine, dosed at 0.25 mg/kg/day divided every 6 hours. If possible, causative medications should be discontinued, while clinicians may alternatively choose to manage the specific side effects with concomitant medication use. Early recognition and treatment of serotonin syndrome generally lead to a favorable prognosis. Prevention should be considered the standard of care in managing these children, through close monitoring of patients who are taking multiple medications with potential adverse interactions [3, 4].

5.1.3 Neuroleptic Malignant Syndrome (NMS)

Neuroleptic malignant syndrome is a rare but potentially life-threatening complication with poorly understood pathophysiology. It is primarily associated with dopamine receptor blockers, potentially disrupting thermoregulation and muscle metabolism. Antipsychotic and antiemetic drugs are the most frequent causative agents. Of note, abrupt cessation of dopaminergic agents and dopamine agonists, such as bromocriptine, ropinirole, and pramipexole, can precipitate NMS.

The clinical presentation of NMS includes hyperpyrexia, muscle rigidity, altered mental status, autonomic dysregulation, dysrhythmias, and profuse diaphoresis. Fevers typically hover around 38 °C but can exceed 40 °C. Hyperthermia arises from increased myocyte metabolic activity and dysregulated hypothalamic thermoregulation. Generalized muscle rigidity presents as consistent resistance throughout all ranges of movement. Autonomic instability may manifest as tachycardia, labile or elevated blood pressure, and tachypnea. Symptoms typically emerge within the first 2 weeks of antipsychotic therapy initiation, though the association with drug usage is idiosyncratic. NMS can ensue following a single dose or long-term treatment with a consistent dosage of the same agent. The occurrence of NMS is not dose-dependent; however, higher doses constitute a risk factor.

Diagnosis of NMS requires laboratory tests to evaluate muscle function and organ damage, which typically reveal elevated creatine kinase levels exceeding 1000 units/L. Other nonspecific laboratory anomalies may include leukocytosis, mild elevations in lactate dehydrogenase, alkaline phosphatase, liver transaminases, and electrolyte imbalances such as hypocalcemia, hypomagnesemia, hypo- and hypernatremia, hyperkalemia, and metabolic acidosis.

NMS management involves immediate cessation of the offending medication. Supportive care entails maintaining cardiorespiratory stability; ensuring euvolemia via intravenous fluid administration; reducing fever with cooling blankets, gastric lavage with ice water, and applying ice packs to the axillae; managing elevated blood pressure; and utilizing benzodiazepines for agitation control. If creatine kinase levels are substantially elevated, high-volume intravenous fluids with urine alkalinization may assist in preventing or alleviating renal failure secondary to rhabdomyolysis [5].

5.1.4 Posterior Reversible Encephalopathy Syndrome (PRES)

Posterior reversible encephalopathy syndrome (PRES) is a clinico-radiographic syndrome with a wide array of underlying etiologies, often linked to disruptions in cerebral autoregulation and endothelial function. The clinical presentation of this syndrome includes headaches, seizures, altered mental status, and visual disturbances, alongside the characteristic presence of white matter abnormalities in the brain. Seizures and particularly status epilepticus are prevalent, with nonconvulsive status epilepticus potentially being more frequent than generalized status epilepticus. Hypertension is the most common precipitating factor in PRES; however, other contributing factors include renal disease, autoimmune disorders, infections, and medications. Certain medications, such as chemotherapeutics, rituximab, tacrolimus, tyrosine kinase inhibitors, carbamazepine, and lithium, have been linked to PRES. It is noteworthy that the threshold for triggering PRES may be at normal therapeutic levels for some patients. Notably, cytotoxic therapies, particularly cyclosporine, have been frequently associated with neurologic manifestations of PRES.

Diagnosing PRES requires a comprehensive evaluation, involving a detailed patient history, a thorough physical examination, and appropriate imaging studies. The fundoscopic examination in PRES patients typically appears normal, while deep tendon reflexes may exhibit brisk responses, and Babinski signs may be present. Neuroimaging, primarily noncontrast CT or MRI, helps confirm the presence of characteristic white matter abnormalities that are predominantly localized in the posterior region of the brain. Magnetic resonance imaging (MRI) typically reveals hyperintense signals on T2-weighted and fluid-attenuated inversion recovery (FLAIR) images, providing valuable diagnostic insights. Immediate management of PRES involves prompt administration of anti-seizure medications, such as benzodiazepines or antiepileptic drugs, followed by control of elevated blood pressure, which is frequently deemed as the precipitating factor. Long-term management strategies may entail adjustments to medications associated with PRES, lifestyle modifications, and regular monitoring of brain function to detect any recurrent episodes or complications [6].

5.2 *Drug-Induced Liver Injury in Pediatric Patients*

Children with complex chronic conditions undergoing treatment with a combination of medications are at higher risk of drug-induced liver injury (DILI) due to drug interactions or genetic predisposition to an idiosyncratic immune response. There are typically three patterns of hepatic damage in DILI, which include hepatitis or hepatocellular, cholestatic, and mixed [7].

Table 2 Commonly implicated agents in drug-induced hepatitis and effects

Medication class	Medications	Clinical effect
Antimicrobial	Minocycline, azithromycin, isoniazid, trimethoprim/sulfa, oxacillin, cefdinir, cefepime, erythromycin, nitrofurantoin, ketoconazole	Hepatitis
Antiepileptic	Valproate, lamotrigine, carbamazepine, ethosuximide, phenobarbital, phenytoin	Hepatitis, cholestasis/ mixed
Antineoplastic	Mercaptopurine, thioguanine, asparaginase, pegaspargase	Hepatitis
Psychotropic	Atomoxetine, methylphenidate, fluoxetine	Hepatitis
Analgesic	Acetaminophen	Hepatitis
Muscle relaxant	Dantrolene	Hepatitis
Anti-inflammatory	Diclofenac	Hepatitis
Antihypertensive	Methyldopa	Hepatitis
Antituberculosis	Pyrazinamide	Hepatitis
Diabetes mellitus, Type 2	Troglitazone	Hepatitis
Miscellaneous	ACE inhibitors, amoxicillin-clavulanic acid, azathioprine, bosentan, chlorpromazine, erythromycin, phenytoin, sulfonamides, sulindac, terbinafine, tricyclic antidepressants	Hepatitis, cholestasis/ mixed

A hepatitis pattern of liver damage, which appears to be the most frequent type of DILI, typically presents acutely, with disease severity ranging from mildly elevated enzymes without symptoms to fulminant liver failure. The most common presenting symptoms in these children include jaundice, fever, and rash. The median value of the laboratory findings at the onset of DILI in the affected children includes alanine aminotransferase (ALT) of 411 U/L, alkaline phosphatase (Alk P) of 203 U/L, and total bilirubin of 3.3 mg/dL. Progressive liver damage may lead to further elevation of these values, with the median peak ALT reaching 732 U/L, Alk P of 288 U/L, and total bilirubin of 4.0 mg/dL. In one study using the data from the DILI network, nearly 17% of these children had persistently abnormal laboratory values up to 6 months following the onset of DILI, suggesting chronic liver changes.

Antimicrobials and antiepileptics are the most frequently associated drug categories, with minocycline and valproate as the most commonly implicated individual medications [8]. Table 2 describes the specific medications and their pathologic effect (Table 2).

5.2.1 Management and Prognosis

Preliminary steps in treating children with DILI include discontinuation of the offending medication and supportive care. Presently, there is insufficient data regarding the efficacy of any treatments to prevent liver failure, mitigate damage, or hasten recovery in children, thus leaving the use of any modalities up to the clinician's empirical clinical judgment. Prompt consultation with a pediatric hepatologist and hospital admission for observation and supportive care of the more severe cases may help optimize these children's treatment course and outcome.

5.3 *Drug-Induced Renal Injury in Pediatric Patients*

Drug-induced renal injury, a significant contributor to kidney failure in pediatric patients, can result in acute or chronic conditions that often lead to lifelong disabilities. Pediatric patients are especially susceptible due to their developing physiology and greater vulnerability to nephrotoxic medications. In a study of patients in the hospital setting, 18–27% of acute kidney injuries were attributed to drug-induced renal injuries, demonstrating its widespread impact [9]. There are six different types of drug-mediated renal injuries including hemodynamically mediated renal failure, glomerulonephritis (GN), acute tubular necrosis (ATN), acute interstitial nephritis (AIN), papillary necrosis (PN), and obstructive nephropathy.

5.3.1 Hemodynamically Mediated Renal Failure

Hemodynamically mediated renal failure results from altered renal blood flow. Medications such as NSAIDs, ACEIs, ARBs, calcineurin inhibitors, and triamterene are key contributors. Clinical manifestations may include decreased urine output, fluid retention, edema, lethargy, dyspnea, and elevated creatinine levels. Management of hemodynamically mediated renal failure typically requires swift recognition of renal dysfunction, appropriate dose adjustment of the causative medications, or complete withdrawal of the offending drug, if indicated. Future preventive measures include careful medication selection and close monitoring of renal function in patients at risk.

5.3.2 Glomerulonephritis (GN)

GN encompasses a wide array of glomerular diseases, including drug-induced forms that can present as various types of renal injury. The clinical spectrum of drug-induced GN is broad, spanning from nephrotic syndrome to focal segmental glomerulosclerosis (FSGS), membranous nephropathy (MN), and membranoproliferative GN. Drugs like NSAIDs, ampicillin, rifampin, foscarnet, and lithium are commonly implicated in drug-induced GN. Management often entails supportive care for extrarenal symptoms and the use of immunosuppressive medications to treat the underlying immune processes.

5.3.3 Acute Tubular Necrosis (ATN)

ATN is an acute kidney injury that arises primarily due to the direct cytotoxic effect of certain medications, most notably aminoglycosides (AG), amphotericin B (AmphoB), radiocontrast dye, and cisplatin. Nephrotoxicity can vary, with clinical manifestations presenting as renal insufficiency, proteinuria, and electrolyte wasting. Prevention and treatment of ATN generally involve dose adjustments, changes in administration methods, or discontinuation of the causative agent. Ongoing research is aimed at developing new therapeutic strategies to minimize the incidence and severity of ATN.

5.3.4 Acute Allergic Interstitial Nephritis (AIN)

AIN is an inflammatory condition affecting the interstitium and tubules of the kidneys, often induced by an allergic reaction to medications. It accounts for 10–15% of drug-induced renal injuries. Common causative medications include antibiotics, particularly penicillin and cephalosporins, and nonsteroidal anti-inflammatory drugs (NSAIDs). Clinical manifestations of AIN are wide-ranging, from fever and skin rash to eosinophilia and various kidney abnormalities. In most cases, discontinuing the drug leads to the resolution of symptoms, although some severe cases may require steroid therapy.

5.3.5 Papillary Necrosis (PN)

Papillary necrosis is frequently associated with analgesic abuse but can also occur due to other underlying medical conditions. Safe and judicious use of analgesics, along with patient education and adequate hydration, is a crucial preventive strategy.

5.3.6 Obstructive Nephropathy

Obstructive nephropathy refers to the obstruction of urine flow resulting from crystallization or sedimentation of certain drugs within the renal tubules. Medications such as acyclovir, sulfadiazine, and methotrexate are primary culprits. Often asymptomatic, some patients may present with nausea, vomiting, and abdominal pain. Preventive measures include slow drug infusion, maintaining patient hydration, and avoiding rapid bolus dosing.

5.3.7 Drug-Induced Diabetes Insipidus

Drug-induced diabetes insipidus is characterized by disruption in the kidneys' ability to resorb and conserve water. This condition may be caused by medications such as lithium, demeclocycline, amphotericin B, ifosfamide, ofloxacin, orlistat, antivirals like cidofovir, and antifungal medications, which may interfere with the

Table 3 Commonly implicated agents in drug-induced renal damage and effects

Renal injury type	Medications
Hemodynamically mediated renal failure	NSAIDs, ACEIs, ARBs, calcineurin inhibitors, triamterene
Nephrotic syndrome	NSAIDs, ampicillin, rifampin, foscarnet, lithium
Focal segmental glomerulosclerosis	Lithium, heroin, pamidronate
Membranous nephropathy	NSAIDs, gold therapy, mercury, penicillamine
Membranoproliferative glomerulonephritis	Hydralazine
Acute tubular injury	Aminoglycosides, amphotericin B, radiocontrast dye, cisplatin
Acute interstitial nephritis	Penicillins, cephalosporins, sulfonamides, fluoroquinolones, vancomycin, omeprazole, pantoprazole
Calcineurin inhibitor nephrotoxicity	Cyclosporin, tacrolimus
Papillary necrosis	NSAIDs, aspirin, acetaminophen
Obstructive nephropathy	Acyclovir, sulfadiazine, methotrexate, triamterene, foscarnet, indinavir

production or action of antidiuretic hormone (ADH). In its mild form, it is relatively common in almost all patients who are sick or have acute or chronic kidney disease. Patients with moderate to severe disease typically present with polyuria (urine output exceeding 2 L/m^2) and nocturia leading to polydipsia and potentially dehydration. Due to disruption in ADH function, which is highest during the night, nocturia may be the earliest warning sign of drug-induced diabetes insipidus.

The diagnosis of drug-induced diabetes insipidus involves evaluation of urine and blood osmolality, as well as antidiuretic hormone (ADH) levels. In untreated patients, the serum sodium levels are typically within the higher end of the normal range, serving as a trigger for thirst to compensate for the excessive loss of water through urine. However, children with impaired thirst function or expression are at increased risk of developing moderate to severe hypernatremia (elevated serum sodium levels). This scenario is particularly observed in patients with central nervous system lesions, who also experience reduced thirst sensation (hypodipsia) or ability to access free water (adipsia) independently [10].

Treatment options include discontinuing the offending medication, replacing fluids and electrolytes, and desmopressin to exert antidiuretic effect. Drug-induced diabetes insipidus may be completely or partially reversed [11] (Table 3).

5.3.8 Management and Prognosis

Effective management of drug-induced renal injury largely depends on early recognition and intervention. The initial step often involves removal or dose reduction of the offending medication. This alone can lead to remission of symptoms, though damage may become irreversible in severe cases. Therefore, vigilance in monitoring is paramount for patients receiving potentially nephrotoxic medications. Certain preventive strategies, such as adequate hydration for patients receiving medications like indinavir, can also play a crucial role in preventing obstructive nephropathy.

5.4 *Cutaneous Complications*

Cutaneous adverse drug reactions (CADRs) pose a significant risk in the medical management of complex pediatric patients, with a wide spectrum of severity ranging from mild skin irritations to potentially life-threatening systemic conditions. Serious reactions, such as anaphylaxis, erythema multiforme, drug rash with eosinophilia and systemic symptoms (DRESS) syndrome, serum sickness-like reaction, Stevens-Johnson syndrome (SJS), and toxic epidermal necrolysis (TEN), may be triggered by commonly prescribed medications such as antibiotics, antiepileptics, nonsteroidal anti-inflammatory drugs, vaccines, and biological agents.

Timely diagnosis in suspected cases of drug eruption is extremely crucial. However clinical resemblance of these cases to viral exanthems, contact dermatitis, or autoimmune conditions often poses a challenge in making the correct diagnosis. It is important to carefully analyze any drug exposure including prescription and over-the-counter drugs, sedatives, infusions, and herbal remedies. The first step in the treatment of any of these conditions is to promptly identify the cause and remove the triggering agents, followed by other possible treatments, if indicated.

5.4.1 Exanthematous Drug Eruptions (EDEs)

EDEs are the most common drug-induced eruptions, comprising nearly 40% of all adverse cutaneous reactions. The rash can appear between 1 and 21 days after the drug exposure, appearing as symmetric, polymorphic, maculopapular, or morbilliform lesions on the truncal area that spread to the extremities, including the palms and soles. It can also appear in areas of pressure or trauma but spares the mucosal surfaces. Patients often describe the rash as pruritic (Fig. 1).

The most common causative agents are antibiotics (penicillin, cephalosporins, sulfonamides), nonsteroidal anti-inflammatory drugs (NSAIDs), antiepileptics

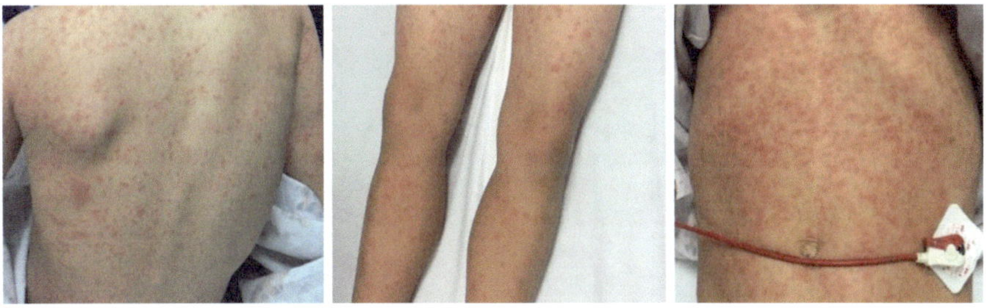

Fig. 1 Examples of exanthematous drug eruptions (EDEs) on the back, legs, and abdomen. Credits: Dr. Carol Cheng

(carbamazepine, hydantoins), and allopurinol. Treatment of EDE consists of stopping the causative medications and prompting systemic administration of antihistamines and corticosteroids [12].

5.4.2 Urticaria

This cutaneous skin reaction represents a type 1 hypersensitivity reaction that causes wheals on the skin and mucous membranes. The rash appears as one or multiple red halos with an edematous center in various sizes that last for 24 hours. Urticaria can accompany angioedema of the lips, eyes, and mucous membranes indicating deep dermal and subcutaneous tissue involvement. This condition can appear as an immediate reaction within 1–2 hours or a delayed reaction of up to several days after drug exposure. Common systemic symptoms include bronchospasms, hypotension, and, in some cases, anaphylaxis. Antibiotics (penicillin, cephalosporins), opioids, aspirin/NSAIDs, and sulfonamides are the most common drugs causing urticaria in children and young adults [13].

While immediate urticarial reactions require discontinuation of the offending drug(s) due to potential anaphylaxis, delayed reactions do not require disruption or change in therapeutics. This rash typically responds to oral or intravenous first- or second-generation antihistamines, while anaphylaxis requires prompt administration of epinephrine and stabilization in an emergency room setting (Fig. 2).

5.4.3 Fixed Drug Eruptions

Fixed drug eruptions (FDEs) are a unique category of cutaneous adverse reactions precipitated by recurrent exposure to a specific drug. Typically, the onset of these reactions is within 24 hours to a several days after re-exposure. In pediatric

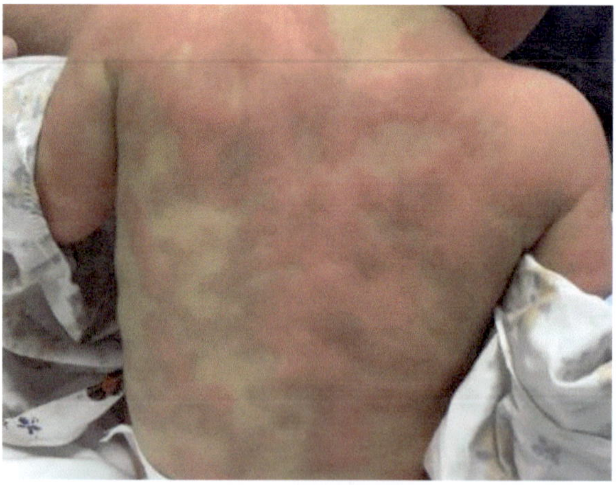

Fig. 2 Example of an urticarial cutaneous reaction. Credits: Dr. Carol Cheng

populations, FDEs commonly manifest as solitary or multiple well-demarcated circular or oval patches, displaying a violaceous hue with the potential to blister or ulcerate. Following the inflammatory phase, the affected site may develop scales or crust formation prior to the peeling stage. This then leads to post-inflammatory hyperpigmentation that is often more prominent in individuals with darker skin types. Although primarily asymptomatic, FDE can induce mild pruritus or discomfort. Known causative agents of FDE include antihistamines (e.g., diphenhydramine, hydroxyzine, loratadine), antibiotics (e.g., amoxicillin, vancomycin, trimethoprim-sulfamethoxazole), nonsteroidal anti-inflammatory drugs (NSAIDs), and anticonvulsants (e.g., phenytoin, phenobarbital). The therapeutic strategy for FDE primarily involves administration of systemic antihistamines or topical corticosteroids [13].

5.4.4 Drug-Induced Hypersensitivity Syndrome (DIHS)/Drug Reaction with Eosinophilia and Systemic Symptoms (DRESS)

DRESS/DIHS is a life-threatening dermatological condition characterized by cutaneous and hematological manifestations, fever, and multi-organ involvement. This condition typically presents 2–6 weeks following drug exposure. Clinical manifestations include pruritic maculopapular exanthem or febrile erythroderma. Approximately 30% of cases demonstrate facial edema, which presents as a periorbital rash that extends caudally. Systemic symptoms may include fever, malaise, cervical lymphadenopathy, and pharyngitis. Multi-organ involvements, including hepatic, pulmonary, cardiac, renal, and pancreatic systems, can lead to prolonged complications. Characteristic laboratory findings include lymphocytosis and eosinophilia. The most frequently implicated agents in DRESS/DIHS are anticonvulsants (e.g., phenytoin, carbamazepine, phenobarbital, lamotrigine), sulfonamides, antibiotics, dapsone, minocycline, allopurinol, and nevirapine. Management of DRESS/DIHS primarily includes corticosteroids (1–2 mg/kg/day) and hospitalization for surveillance and supportive care [13, 14].

5.4.5 Stevens-Johnson Syndrome/Toxic Epidermal Necrolysis

SJS and TEN represent severe and potentially fatal dermatological reactions, with a mortality rate approximating 25%. These conditions typically manifest around 21 days post-drug exposure, initially presenting as erythematous lesions or pruritic macules that progressively coalesce into painful blisters, involving at least two mucosal regions (oral, ocular, and genital). The reaction begins on the face and spreads caudally. Nikolsky's sign can be positive. Systemic symptoms may include fever, malaise, and upper respiratory manifestations. Tachypnea and hypoxia could indicate underlying bronchial tree necrosis and is strongly associated with poor prognosis. SJS and TEN are differentiated based on the extent of skin involvement: SJS affects approximately 10% of the total body surface area,

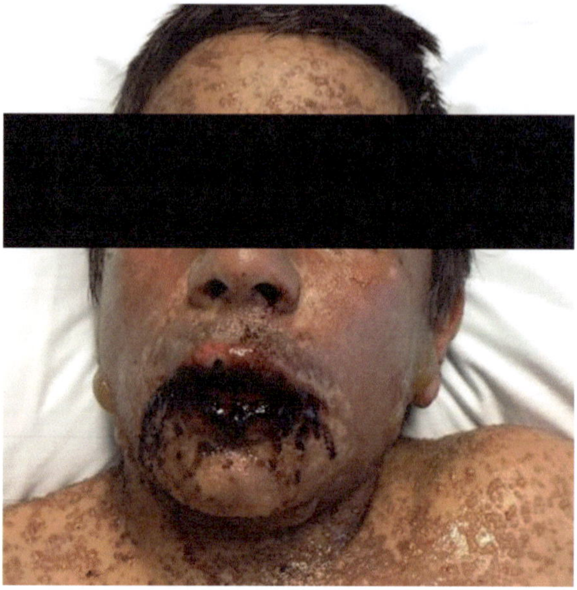

Fig. 3 Example of Steven-Johnson syndrome. Credits: Dr. Carol Cheng

TEN affects over 30%, and SJS-TEN overlap syndrome involves between 10% and 30%. Commonly implicated agents include antiepileptic drugs (e.g., phenytoin, carbamazepine), antibiotics (e.g., sulfonamides, penicillin), NSAIDs, and allopurinol. All suspected cases of SJS and TEN warrant immediate hospitalization for intravenous fluid replenishment, electrolyte management, analgesia, and comprehensive supportive care [13, 14] (Fig. 3).

5.4.6 Acute Generalized Exanthematous Pustulosis (AGEP)

Acute generalized exanthematous pustulosis is a rare, severe cutaneous adverse reaction with an estimated incidence of 1–5 cases per million individuals annually. The rash typically manifests within a span of 24 hours to 4 days following drug exposure. It typically presents as an abrupt onset of erythematous rash featuring small pustules that are primarily found in the axillary or inguinal folds. The lesions coalesce and the begin to desquamate superficiaally. The rash is pruritic or burning and can be, accompanied by fever and leukocytosis. Antibiotics, specifically penicillin and macrolides, are the most common causative agents of AGEP. The management of AGEP primarily involves the use of topical corticosteroids [14] (Table 4).

Table 4 Skin reaction types and causative drugs

Eruption type	Presentation	Systemic symptoms	Causative drugs
Exanthematous	Symmetric, polymorphic maculopapular, or morbilliform lesions	Pruritus	Antibiotics (penicillin, cephalosporins, sulfonamides), nonsteroidal anti-inflammatory drugs (NSAIDs), antiepileptics (carbamazepine, hydantoins), allopurinol
Urticaria	Red halo with an edematous center	Anaphylaxis (bronchospasm, hypotension, syncope)	Antibiotics (penicillin, cephalosporins), opioids, aspirin/NSAIDs, sulfonamides
Fixed drug eruptions	Erythematous-violaceous patch in the same location as drug exposure		Antihistamines (diphenhydramine, hydroxyzine, loratadine), antibiotics (amoxicillin, vancomycin, TMP-SMX), NSAIDs, anticonvulsants (phenytoin, phenobarbital)
Drug-induced hypersensitivity/ DRESS	Pruritic maculopapular exanthem with organ involvement	Fever, lymphadenopathy, lymphocytosis, eosinophilia, arthralgia	Anticonvulsants (phenytoin, carbamazepine, phenobarbital, lamotrigine), sulfonamides, antibiotics, dapsone, minocycline, allopurinol, and nevirapine
Stevens-Johnson syndrome/toxic epidermal necrolysis	Skin blisters arising from erythematous macules in central distribution	Fever, malaise, upper respiratory symptoms	Antiepileptic drugs (phenytoin, carbamazepine), antibiotics (sulfonamides, penicillin), NSAIDs, and allopurinol
Acute generalized exanthematous pustulosis	Abrupt pustular rash that arises in the skin folds	Pruritus, burning, fever, pustulosis with leukocytosis	Antibiotics (penicillin, macrolides)

6 Review Questions

1. A 14-year-old child with medical complexity admitted for feeding intolerance develops facial tics and lip smacking after receiving a medication. Which of the following medications is the most likely causative agent?
   (A) Sertraline
   (B) Omeprazole
   (C) Metoclopramide
   (D) Tacrolimus
2. A 7-year-old patient receiving penicillin for streptococcal pharyngitis develops a renal complication of the medication. Which of the following is the most likely mechanism of renal injury?

(A) Allergic interstitial nephritis
(B) Glomerulonephritis
(C) Obstructive nephropathy
(D) Papillary necrosis

3. A 6-year-old female with intractable epilepsy was started on a new medication for seizure control 5 weeks ago. She develops a morbilliform rash, fevers, pharyngitis, and an acute elevation in her liver function tests. Which of the following is the most likely explanation for the findings?

(A) Stevens-Johnson syndrome
(B) Fixed drug eruption
(C) Toxic epidermal necrolysis
(D) Drug reaction with eosinophilia and systemic symptoms (DRESS)

7 Answers

1. **C**. The patient has symptoms concerning for tardive dyskinesia; dopamine receptor-blocking agents such as metoclopramide are the most likely culprits.
2. **A**. The most likely cause of penicillin-related renal complications is acute allergic interstitial nephritis; the other options are not common with penicillin.
3. **D**. The morbilliform rash and multisystem involvement several weeks after starting a new antiepileptic medication are concerning for DRESS; prompt cessation of the new medication is imperative.

8 Takeaway Points

1. Awareness and prevention of adverse drug reactions are critical to the management of children with medical complexity.
2. Complications are even more likely when patients are prescribed multiple medications at once due to drug-drug interactions, including serotonin syndrome and others.
3. Common organ systems involved in adverse drug reactions include neurologic, hepatic, renal, and dermatologic.

References

1. Jain KK. Drug-induced disorders of memory and dementia. In: Drug-induced neurological disorders. Cham: Springer; 2021. p. 11–26.
2. Sachdev PS. Tardive dyskinesia in children: a systematic review. J Paediatr Child Health. 2019;55(2):128–32. https://doi.org/10.1111/jpc.14261.

3. Prakash S, Patel V, Patel S. Serotonin syndrome in children: a review. Indian J Pediatr. 2019;86(7):627–32. https://doi.org/10.1007/s12098-019-02902-1.
4. Godinho EM, Thompson AE, Bramble DJ. Neuroleptic withdrawal versus serotonergic syndrome in an 8-year-old child. J Child Adolesc Psychopharmacol. 2002;12:265.
5. Papolos DF, Teicher MH, Faedda GL. The spectrum of neuroleptic malignant syndrome in children and adolescents. J Child Adolesc Psychopharmacol. 2013;23(3):139–46.
6. Sudulagunta SR, Sodalagunta MB, Kumbhat M, Settikere Nataraju A. Posterior reversible encephalopathy syndrome (PRES). Oxf Med Case Rep. 2017;2017(4):omx011. https://doi.org/10.1093/omcr/omx011.
7. Nathwani RA, Kaplowitz N. Drug hepatotoxicity. Clin Liver Dis. 2006;10(2):207–17, vii. https://doi.org/10.1016/j.cld.2006.05.009.
8. DiPaola F, Molleston JP, Gu J, Cirulli ET, Chalasani N, Barnhart H, Kleiner DE, Hoofnagle JH, Fontana RJ, US Drug Induced Liver Injury Network. Antimicrobials and Antiepileptics Are the Leading Causes of Idiosyncratic Drug-induced Liver Injury in American Children. J Pediatr Gastroenterol Nutr. 2019;69(2):152–9. https://doi.org/10.1097/MPG.0000000000002383.
9. Taber SS, Pasko DA. The epidemiology of drug-induced disorders: the kidney. Expert Opin Drug Saf. 2008;7(6):679–90. https://doi.org/10.1517/14740330802410462.
10. Garofeanu CG, Weir M, Rosas-Arellano MP, et al. Causes of reversible nephrogenic diabetes insipidus: a systematic review. Am J Kidney Dis. 2005;45:626.
11. Bendz H, Aurell M. Drug-induced diabetes insipidus: incidence, prevention and management. Drug Saf. 1999;21(6):449–56. https://doi.org/10.2165/00002018-199921060-00002. PMID: 10612269.
12. Heelan K, Shear NH. Cutaneous drug reactions in children: an update. Pediatr Drugs. 2013;15:493–503. https://doi.org/10.1007/s40272-013-0039-z.
13. Al Aboud DM, Nessel TA, Hafsi W. Cutaneous adverse drug reaction. [Updated 2023 Apr 10]. In: StatPearls [Internet]. Treasure Island: StatPearls Publishing; 2023 Jan-. Available from: https://www.ncbi.nlm.nih.gov/books/NBK533000/.
14. Mockenhaupt M. Severe drug-induced skin reactions: clinical pattern, diagnostics and therapy. J Dtsch Dermatol Ges. 2009;7:142–62. https://doi.org/10.1111/j.1610-0387.2008.06878.x.

Index

A
Abdominal organ perforation, 148
Abdominal pseudocyst formation, 148
Absolute neutrophil count, 17
Acute bronchiolitis, 82, 83
Acute generalized exanthematous pustulosis (AGEP), 202
Acute lymphoid leukemia, 15, 16
Acute rejection (ACR), 186
Acute tubular necrosis (ATN), 197
Adrenal insufficiency (AI), 27
Adrenal steroidogenesis pathway, 28
Adrenocorticotrophic hormone (ACTH), 28–30
Adverse drug reactions (ADRs), 190
  See also Polypharmacy
Airway clearance therapy (ACT), 73
Albuterol, 83
Allergic interstitial nephritis (AIN), 197
Allogenic hematopoietic stem cell transfer, 60
Antegrade colonic enema (ACE), 131
Antidiuretic effect, 198
Antidiuretic hormone (ADH), 28, 198
Antiepileptics, 195
Antimicrobials, 195
Antipseudomonal beta-lactam, 18
Appendicitis, 18
Atopy, 83

B
Baclofen withdrawal syndrome, 66
11-Beta-hydroxylase deficiency, 30
Bi-level positive airway pressure (BiPAP), 83
Bladder perforation, 135
Bladder reconstruction
  CCC, 133–135
  complications, 135, 136
  CT cystogram, 135, 137
  differential diagnosis, 135
  patient history, 131, 132
  VP shunt, 136
Blalock-Thomas-Taussig (BTT) shunt, 46
Blood pressure (BP), 43, 49
  See also Kidney transplantation
Bronchopulmonary dysplasia (BPD), 81, 82
B-type natriuretic peptide (BNP), 185

C
Cardiogenic shock, 84
Cardiomyopathy (CMY), 158
Catheter malposition, 124
Catheter related thrombosis (CRT), 123, 124
Central (secondary) adrenal insufficiency (CAI), 28, 29
Central line
  blood cultures, 123
  breakage, 122
  catheter malposition, 124
  CLABSIs, 124, 125
  complications, 122
  CRT, 123, 124
  CVC, 122
  dressing changes, 124
  patient history, 121, 122
  photos, 126
  PPE, 124
  repair kit, 123
  silastic tunneled catheters, 123

A. Kamzan et al. (eds.), *Children with Medical Complexity in the Emergency Department*, https://doi.org/10.1007/978-3-031-62517-6

Central line-associated blood stream infection (CLABSI), 97, 124
Central venous catheter (CVC), 122–124
Cerebrospinal fluid (CSF), 142, 143, 145
  epidemiology and timing, 145
  management, 147, 148
  microbiology, 146
  pathogenesis, 145, 146
  risk factors, 145
  shunts, 65
  signs and symptoms, 146
  work-up and diagnosis, 147
Children with medical complexity (CMC), 1, 2
  CSF shunt, 65
  development, 64
  differential diagnosis, 64
  intrathecal baclofen, 65, 66
  patient history, 63, 64
  symptoms, 66
Cholangitis, 180
Cholecystitis, 18
Chronic lung disease (CLD), 81, 82, 85
Clean intermittent catheterization (CIC), 133
Congenital adrenal hyperplasia (CAH), 27, 28, 30
Congenital heart disease (CHD), 158
  clinical presentation and differential diagnosis, 47–49
  management, 49, 50
  pathophysiology and epidemiology, 45–47
  patient history, 43–45
Continent catheterizable channels (CCC), 133–135
Continuous positive airway pressure (CPAP), 83
Corticosteroids, 59
Creatinine, 173
Crohn disease, 95
Cutaneous adverse drug reactions (CADRs)
  AGEP, 202
  definition, 199
  diagnosis and intervention, 199
  DRESS/DIHS, 201
  EDEs, 199, 200
  FDEs, 200, 201
  SJS and TEN, 201, 202
  urticaria, 200
Cutibacterium acnes, 146
Cystic fibrosis (CF)
  ACT, 73
  CFTR, 72–74
  life-threatening complications, 74
  patient history, 71, 72
  pneumothorax, 74
  pulmonary exacerbations, 73, 74
Cystic fibrosis transmembrane conductance regulator (CFTR), 72–74
Cytomegalovirus (CMV), 179

D
Deep venous thromboses (DVT), 123
Dialysate fluid, 36
Diarrhea, 96, 173
Dilated cardiomyopathy (DCM), 158–159
Direct laryngoscopy and bronchoscopy (DLB), 105
D-lactic acid, 97
Drug-induced diabetes insipidus, 197, 198
Drug-induced hypersensitivity syndrome (DIHS)/Drug reaction with eosinophilia and systemic symptoms (DRESS), 201
Drug-induced liver injury (DILI), 194–196
Drug-induced renal injury
  AIN, 197
  ATN, 197
  drug-induced diabetes insipidus, 197, 198
  glomerulonephritis, 196
  hemodynamically mediated renal failure, 196
  management and prognosis, 198
  obstructive nephropathy, 197
  papillary necrosis, 197
  types, 196
Ductus arteriosus, 84
Dysautonomia, 66

E
Edema, 172
Effusion, 47
Emergency department (ED), 1
Emergency information forms (EIFs), 2, 3
Endomyocardial biopsy (EMB), 160
End stage renal disease (ESRD), 170
  hemodialysis, 36
  peritoneal dialysis, 35–39
Enteral feeding tubes, 116, 117
Enterobacter, 180
Epstein Barr Virus (EBV), 179
Exanthematous drug eruptions (EDEs), 199, 200

F
F508del mutation, 75
Febrile neutropenia, 17–20
Fever, 55, 57, 59
  SBS (*see* Short bowel syndrome (SBS))

See also Neutropenia fever
Fixed drug eruptions (FDEs), 200, 201
Fluid resuscitation, 38, 99, 155
Fontan procedure, 47

G
Gastrostomy tube (G-tube)
de-clog, 118
dislodgement, 117, 118
drainage, 117
enteral feeding, 116, 117
granulation tissue, 117
movement of, 117
patient history, 115, 116
peristomal leakage, 117
Glenn obstruction, 48
Glenn procedure, 43, 46
Glomerulonephritis (GN), 196
Glucocorticoids, 29, 171, 172
Granulation tissue, 106, 117
G-tube, 98
Guidelines for Ruling out and Assessing Source of Pain (GRASP), 64, 66
Gut ischemia, 48

H
Healthcare system, 2
Heart transplantation
CHD, 158
patient history, 157, 158
post-transplantation, 159
rejection
clinical presentation, 160
differential diagnosis, 161
initial management, 163
initial workup, 162
pathophysiology and timing, 159, 160
Heat-and-moisture exchange (HME), 107
Hemodialysis (HD), 36
Hemodynamically mediated renal failure, 196
Hemophagocytic lymphohistiocytosis (HLH)
anemia and thrombocytopenia, 59
bicytopenia, 57
bone marrow biopsy and flow cytometry, 58–59
diagnostic criteria, 58
ferritin, 58
immune hyperactivation, 56
Kawasaki disease, 59
management, 59, 60
patient history, 55, 56
persistent fever, 57
rheumatologic disorder, 57
trigger, 57
Hemoptysis, 74
Hepatic artery thrombosis, 179
Hepatomegaly, 57
High flow nasal cannula (HFNC), 83
Human leukocyte antigens (HLA), 159
21-Hydroxylase deficiency, 30
17-Hydroxyprogesterone (17OHP), 27
Hyperacute rejection, 159
Hyperammonemia, 7
Hyperchloremic metabolic acidosis, 135
Hypertension, 59, 172, 194
Hypoplastic aortic arch, 43
Hypoplastic left heart syndrome (HLHS), 43, 45
Hypotension, 86
Hypothalamic-pituitary-adrenal axis, 27

I
Ileal pouch-anal anastomosis (IPAA), 151, 152
Immunosuppressants, 161
Inborn errors of metabolism (IEM)
clinical presentation, 7, 8
complications and comorbiditics, 10, 11
history, 5, 6
initial evaluation and management, 8–10
metabolic crisis, 7
Inferior cavopulmonary connection, 47
Inferior vena cava (IVC), 47
Inhaled nitric oxide (iNO), 48
Intestinal failure associated liver disease (IFALD), 97
Intestinal transplantation, 185
Intralipids, 10
Intrathecal baclofen (ITB), 65, 66
Irritability, 64–66

K
Kawasaki disease, 59
Kidney transplantation
complications, 171
dialysis, 170
diarrhea, 173
edema, 172
electrolytes, 173
glomerular filtration rate, 174
hypertension, 172
immunosuppression, 171
initial management, 173
patient history, 169, 170
side effects, 171

L
Lactate dehydrogenase, 58
Lactated Ringer's (LR), 98
Length of stay (LOS), 83
Linezolid, 180
Liver transplantation
  acute rejection, 179, 180
  central line, 180
  EBV and CMV, 179
  history, 177, 178
  intra-abdominal infections, 180
  laboratory findings, 179, 180
  PTLD, 178, 179
  work-up, 180
Lung parenchymal diseases, 84

M
Macrophage activation syndrome (MAS), 57
Mechanical ventilation, 83, 86
Methylenedioxymethamphetamine (MDMA), 192
Mineralocorticoid deficiency, 30
Mitrofanoff procedure, 133, 135
Monti procedure, 133
Mycophenolate mofetil, 171

N
Nebulized hypertonic saline, 83
Necrotizing enterocolitis (NEC), 48
Neuroleptic malignant syndrome (NMS), 193, 194
Neutropenia fever, 21
Neutropenic fever, 16–18, 20
Nikolsky's sign, 201
Non-infectious complications, 143, 144
Non-steroidal anti-inflammatory drugs (NSAIDs), 174
Norwood procedure, 46

O
Obstructive nephropathy, 197
Ornithine transcarbamylase deficiency, 5
Oro-bucco-lingual region, 192
Ostomy
  complications, 153, 154
  double-barrel colostomy, 153
  high output fluid loss, 155
  loop and end ileostomies, 153
  loop colostomy, 153
  parastomal hernia, 154
  parastomal infection, 155
  patient history, 151, 152
  peristomal skin problems, 154
  signs and symptoms, 152
  stoma, 152, 153
  stomal necrosis, 154
  stomal retraction, 154
  stomal stenosis, 154
Oxygen supplementation, 49, 50, 82

P
Palivizumab, 86, 87
Papillary necrosis (PN), 197
Parastomal hernia, 154
Parenteral nutrition (PN), 95, 97
Paroxysmal sympathetic hyperactivity (PSH), 66
Patent ductus arteriosus (PDA), 46
Peripherally inserted central catheter (PICC), 122
Peristomal leakage, 117
Peritoneal dialysis (PD)
  antibiotics, 38, 39
  catheter, 37
  cause of, 37
  diagnostic criteria, 38
  inpatient vs outpatient treatment, 39
  patient history, 35, 36
  quality of life, 37
  signs and symptoms, 38
Persistent pulmonary hypertension (PPHN), 83
Personal protective equipment (PPE), 124
Pneumothorax, 74, 85, 86
Polypharmacy
  CADRs
    AGEP, 202
    definition, 199
    diagnosis and intervention, 199
    DRESS/DIHS, 201
    EDEs, 199, 200
    FDEs, 200, 201
    SJS and TEN, 201, 202
    urticaria, 200
  DILI, 194–196
  drug-induced renal injury
    AIN, 197
    ATN, 197
    drug-induced diabetes insipidus, 197, 198
    glomerulonephritis, 196

hemodynamically mediated renal failure, 196
management and prognosis, 198
obstructive nephropathy, 197
papillary necrosis, 197
types, 196
neurologic complications
NMS, 193, 194
PRES, 194
serotonin syndrome, 192, 193
symptoms, 190, 191
tardive dyskinesia, 191, 192
patient history, 189, 190
skin reaction types and causative drugs, 203
Posterior reversible encephalopathy syndrome (PRES), 161, 194
Post-transplant lymphoproliferative disorder (PTLD), 161, 178, 179
Prematurity
acute bronchiolitis, 82, 83
bronchopulmonary dysplasia, 81, 82
patient history, 79, 80
PHC, 83–85
pneumothorax, 85, 86
RSV injection, 86, 87
Primary adrenal insufficiency (PAI), 27, 29
Pseudomonas aeruginosa, 73, 180
Pulmonary arterial hypertension (PAH), 48
Pulmonary exacerbations, 73, 74
Pulmonary hypertension, 84–85
Pulmonary hypertensive crisis (PHC), 83–85
Pulmonary vascular resistance (PVR), 83

R
Rash, 57
Recurrent pulmonary exacerbations, 71
Renal failure, 59
Residual renal function, 38
Respiratory distress syndrome, *see* Prematurity
Respiratory syncytial virus (RSV), 82
Rett syndrome, 192
Rhabdomyolysis, 66
Rheumatologic disorder, 57
Right upper quadrant (RUQ), 177

S
Seizures, 59
Sepsis, 185
Serial transverse enteroplasty procedure (STEP), 96
Serotonin syndrome (SS), 192, 193
Short bowel syndrome (SBS)
CLABSI, 97
clinical outcome, 99
diarrhea, 96
differential diagnosis, 98
D-lactate, 97
etiology, 95
gastrointestinal symptoms, 96
intestinal adaptation, 96
management, 98
parenteral nutrition, 95–97
patient history, 93–95
SIBO, 97
Shunt malfunctions, 144, 146
Silastic tunneled catheters, 123
Small bowel transplantation (SBT)
ACR, 185, 186
biomarkers, 185
chronic rejection, 185
electrolytes, 186
intestinal transplant, 185
patient history, 183, 184
sepsis, 185
solid-organ transplants, 184
Small intestinal bacterial overgrowth syndrome (SIBO), 97
Splenomegaly, 57
Sputum culture, 74
Staphylococcus aureus, 74, 146
Stevens-Johnson Syndrome/Toxic Epidermal Necrolysis (SJS/TEN), 201, 202
Stomal necrosis, 154
Stomal retraction, 154
Stomal stenosis, 154
Suction trauma, 106, 107
Superior cavopulmonary connection, 46
Suprapubic catheter (SPC), 135, 136
Synagis, 86
Systemic arterial pressure, 83
Systemic outflow obstruction, 48

T
Tachycardia, 98, 172
Tacrolimus toxicity, 161, 173
Tardive dyskinesia (TD), 191, 192
Telehealth, 1
Thrombocytopenia, 59
Thrombus, 47
Total proctocolectomy (TPC), 152
Tracheal bleeding, 106
Tracheal stenosis, 108

Tracheo-innominate artery fistula
        (TIF), 108–110
Tracheostomy tube
    catastrophic tube-related events, 108–110
    cuffs, 107, 108
    definition, 104, 105
    epidemiology, 104, 105
    patient history, 103, 104
    tracheal secretions, blood in, 105–107
Trans-appendicular continent cystostomy, 133
Traumatic brain injury (TBI)
    adrenal insufficiency, 27–30
    clinical history, 26
    patient history, 25, 26
Triglycerides, 58
Typhlitis, 18

U
Ulcerative colitis (UC), 151
Urinary tract infections (UTI), 134, 172
Urticaria, 200

V
Vancomycin, 18, 180
Venous thromboembolism (VTE), 123
Ventriculoperitoneal (VP) shunt, 135
    complications, 148
    components, 142
    CSF, 142, 143, 145
        epidemiology and timing, 145
        management, 147, 148
        microbiology, 146
        pathogenesis, 145, 146
        risk factors, 145
        signs and symptoms, 146
        work-up and diagnosis, 147
    non-infectious complications, 143, 144
    patient history, 141, 142
Vesicular monoamine transporter type 2
        inhibitors (VMAT2), 192
Vitamin B12 deficiency, 134

MIX
Papier aus verantwortungsvollen Quellen
Paper from responsible sources
FSC® C105338

If you have any concerns about our products,
you can contact us on
ProductSafety@springernature.com

In case Publisher is established outside the EU,
the EU authorized representative is:
Springer Nature Customer Service Center GmbH
Europaplatz 3, 69115 Heidelberg, Germany

Printed by Libri Plureos GmbH
in Hamburg, Germany